Mak[...]
in the Wellness
Industry

Make a Fortune in the Wellness Industry

How to Initiate, Participate and Profit from the Trillion Dollar Wellness Healthcare Revolution

Selva Sugunendran

CEng, MIEE, MCMI, CHt, MIMDHA, MBBNLP

#1 Best Selling Author, Speaker & Coach

Medical Disclaimer: The author of this book is a competent, experienced writer.

He has taken every opportunity to ensure all information presented here is correct and up to date at the time of writing. No documentation within this book has been evaluated by the Food and Drug Administration, and no documentation should be used to diagnose, treat, cure, or prevent any disease.

Any information is to be used for educational and information purposes only. It should never be substituted for the medical advice from your own doctor or other health care professionals.

We do not dispense medical advice, prescribe drugs or diagnose any illnesses with our literature.

The author and publisher are not responsible or liable for any self or third party diagnosis made by visitors based upon the content in this book. Neither does the author or publisher in any way endorse any commercial products or services linked from other websites to this book.

Please, always consult your doctor or health care specialist if you are in any way concerned about your physical wellbeing.

This book was printed in the United States of America.

First Printing: 2012

To order additional copies of this book, contact:

Xlibris Corporation

0-800-644-6988

www.xlibrispublishing.co.uk

Orders@Xlibrispublishing.co.uk

303966

CONTENTS

DEDICATION

This book is dedicated to my late mother, Violet Ratnam, whose efforts to seek, find and implement preventive solutions to avert the constant Asthmatic attacks I had during my childhood instilled in me the importance of always looking for preventive measures rather than treatment after the fact.

This book is dedicated to her memory. I love you and miss you Amma (Mom)

ACKNOWLEDGEMENTS

I WOULD LIKE TO acknowledge the following great men who have inspired me and whose contributions to the Wellness solutions have indeed encouraged me to write this book so that more people will be able to lead healthier, happier and longer lives, while becoming wealthier and successful in the process.

J.I. Rodale, the man who in my opinion, paved the way for the start of the drive from "Sickness based to Wellness based Solutions". We will remember him as the man who put his entire wealth at risk to fight for the great change towards "Wellness solutions".

Dr. James L Chestnut, the master of "evidence-based . . . argument for lifestyle intervention as the foundation of Wellness".

Steve Demos, often referred to as "The Soy Wonder". His search for a product that required no customer education but containing "freshness, familiarity, and convenience" gave us the Silk soymilk that soon opened the doors for millions of people to the healthy milk alternative".

Carl F. Rehnborg, Inventor of Multivitamins, who successfully used technology to solve the problems that had been created by processed and fast-food industries.

Frank Yanowitz, The Wellness Cardiologist, whose understanding of the connections between diet, exercise and health has helped many to take better care of their heart as well as their general health.

Paul Zane Pilzer, the world-renowned economist, a visionary, a multimillionaire software entrepreneur, and the author of eight best-selling books. I have read all his books and feel enlightened by his contribution to the world at large. I first read his book, "God Wants You to Be Rich: The Theology of Economics". Since then I have read all his books including, "The Wellness Revolution", "The Next Millionaires" and "The New Health Insurance Solution". I must admit that his foresight, understanding and strength of character to stand firm on his belief to bring about necessary changes, has enriched my life and energized me to write this book with full conviction.

Most importantly, I wish to give thanks to my family. I thank my wife for her support and understanding as I spent long hours researching and travelling to gather the required data to write this book. My thanks go to my mother for instilling in me the importance of prevention over treatment and my father for teaching the disciplines necessary to take on and be successful in any challenge I undertook. I would also acknowledge my grandmother for instilling in me the great Christian values of loving, caring, giving and sharing, in addition to learning to protect my honesty and integrity at all times. These have become my core values and beliefs.

My thanks also go to my son Shaun and daughter (in-law), Florence, for giving and sharing the love and joy of my two grandchildren, Jason and Lisa. Jason, at just 5 years old, also provides the inspiration I need with his creativity, positive outlook and analytical mind.

And, of course, thank you to Ann McIndoo, who assisted me through the process of editing this book. My thanks also go to my lovely niece Samantha Manoharan for checking my articles.

I would also like to thank Martin Read, Rex Thorne, Fred Jane, Alan Clasby, Brian Tracy, Peggy McColl, Stephanie J Hale and Phill Turner for their contribution, at various stages of my life, to my own personal development.

My grateful thanks go to those who have inspired me during my journey including Pastor T.U Thomas, Dr. Paul Gnanayutham and Dr Topher Morrison.

My special heartfelt thanks go to all I have mentioned, and to those I couldn't mention too. You know who you are!.

I cannot end this acknowledgement without giving thanks to God who has provided me with everything I need as illustrated in Philippians 4:verses 11-13.

In this Book, You Will Learn About

* The Current Unsustainable "Sickness-Based" Healthcare System

* The Wellness Alternative: Preventive Healthcare Solutions

* How To Profit From the New Opportunity of the One Trillion Dollar Industry in the Making

The healthcare industry in the United States is getting ready to undergo a major revision. The fundamental paradigm of care will shift from treating those who are already sick to adopting new models of preventative care to help those who are still well and want to stay that way. This is a revolutionary change to healthcare that is going to save the country billions of dollars in revenue.

Believe me, that revenue isn't just going to disappear. It's going to change hands. And if you follow the instructions I've set forth in this book, those hands could be yours!

This book is all about seeing what's happening in our world and using our creative minds to make a profit from it. I've done it before, I've seen it done, and I know you can do it because I'm here to help you. All you have to do is believe in yourself, grasp this golden opportunity and soon you'll be profiting more than you ever dreamed possible from the Wellness revolution.

To Your Success!

Selva

Selva Sugunendran,
CEng, MIEE, MCMI, CHt, MIMDHA, MBBNLP
#1 Best Selling Author, Speaker & Coach

INTRODUCTION

I'M IN THE *business of success. While I've run different types of businesses over the years and filled just about every position you could imagine, my real passion is success. By that I mean the act of succeeding. I like to do it. I like to see others do it. Perhaps more than anything else, I like to teach others how to be successful.*

Success is all about getting from where you are in life to where you want to be, and that's what this book is about. There are rare moments in our lives when the winds of society and culture change in such a way that each and every one of us is granted a pure golden opportunity to grab the reins and achieve total success in our own lives.

Unfortunately, some of us don't recognize the chance until it's come and gone, and once it's gone, it's too late.

I'm writing this because I've seen "the next big thing" coming down the pipe and I want to let you, my friends, know about it.

Well, I'm excited to get started. Shall we?

Selva

CHAPTER ONE

The Current "Sickness-Based" Healthcare System

T HE CONCEPT OF Wellness is not some New Age health trend. Wellness is a fully realized legitimate concept that is, sadly, little discussed in today's healthcare system. When people talk about 'feeling good' or 'feeling healthy', they most simply mean that they feel good physically or that they are not physically showing any signs of sickness or disease.

This is not Wellness.

Wellness encompasses more than our physical self. Wellness is a rich and dynamic perception that encompasses several dimensions. While this may seem confusing at first glance, it really isn't. Basically, Wellness is about being the healthiest possible being in body, mind, and spirit. Wellness is when one's own potential is fully realized and illnesses are not just treatment after the fact.

The dimensions of self that Wellness focuses on are:

- Emotional
- Mental
- Physical
- Social

- Spiritual
- Environmental

When these six dimensions work together and are in harmony they all attribute to Wellness.

I know you're thinking that this sounds completely different than what you thought "being well" meant. The modern concept of "being well" and being healthy is focused on only one dimension, the physical. Think of it this way, we are more than just a physical manifestation of an entity.

We think, create, interact, and laugh; we are a package of many different components. Why focus on just one of those components? Would you only worry about your car's washer fluid and forsake the tires, oil, and everything else that is instrumental to make that car run smoothly? Of course, not. So why forsake your environment or your intellect or your social and spiritual needs to only focus on the physical? It just does not make any sense.

To be healthy, truly healthy with a good sense of Wellness, you must focus on all six of these dimensions. In addition to physical health, Wellness is about "enrich[ing] your life emotionally, reach[ing] more of your potential professionally, improv[ing] your profits financially, and most importantly . . . mak[ing] a greater contribution socially".[1]

---

[1]   Hoffman, Bob, & Deitch, J. (2007). *Discover Wellness: How Staying Healthy Can Make You Rich.* Eagan, MN: Center Path Publishing, p. xii.

Let's take a quick look at these six dimensions before we move on. Maybe by understanding a bit more about the individual parts of Wellness you will be better able to understand how important Wellness is to realizing a healthier and happier you.

Emotional

Stressed out at work? At your wits end at home? Too busy? Over taxed? Over stretched? Sure you are. You are a modern human. Emotional Wellness focuses on handling stress in a healthy manner and not after you had your nervous breakdown.

Mental

When was the last time you created something? Maybe as a child you used to draw or write, but what about now? When did you learn something new just for the sake of learning? Mental Wellness focuses on being mentally active and flexing your imagination and creativity.

Physical

We all have an idea about this one. It is to make sure our body is performing efficiently and is healthy. Avoiding harmful substances and choosing good lifestyle choices all work towards physical Wellness.

Social

Hang out with friends. Take time out of your busy schedule to spend time with your family and the ones you hold dear. Go out into the world and make a difference in someone's life. Do not simply sit behind a computer screen staring dully into that blue glow. Interact with real people!

Spiritual

This is not about theology or which 'Good Book' you subscribe to. This is about your own moral beliefs, ethics, and convictions and making sure that they are healthy.

Environmental

We are our environment. If our environment is sick; so too are we.

By working on all these dimensions in harmony, we can approach a being of true Wellness. This is a state of being that is not dependent upon pill bottles or medical attention as soon as a problem arises.

This is a state of being where we feel good in body, mind, and spirit and focus on the Wellness of Self. Wellness is not some stagnant state you maintain before flu season comes around. Wellness is not a pit stop in between being sick and feeling bad. Wellness is a way of life.

Wellness is the only way of life and it is about time that everyone starts living it.

The State of Affairs with Healthcare

At present, Wellness is not the focus of the current healthcare system in the United States. Don't agree with me? That's understandable. The current healthcare system is so ingrained in the nation's conscience that not too many people really stop to think about how it actually works. It is common knowledge that, "When you get sick, you go to the doctor." On the surface, that seems to make sense, but for some reason we never seem to stop and ask the fundamental question, "Why get sick at all?"

The majority of healthcare facilities are owned and operated by private companies and organizations. They make their money by treating the sick. If a preventive measure to healthcare were to take place, how then would these companies make money?

Pharmaceutical companies alone would stand to lose an untold amount of money if we were to move to a healthcare system based on Wellness and prevention instead of treating symptoms and conditions as they arise.

What it takes is for us, as a society, to dedicate ourselves to the idea of true Wellness, and as Americans, we surely have this potential for greatness in us.

But for now, the way the current system works is simply flawed. We've all been there, in the ER at 3:00 a.m. waiting in a crowded room with the coughing and sneezing masses shuddering with the flu and who knows what else. When we see the doctor they run a few tests, take our temperature and then prescribe some medicine. We are sent on our way and chances are no one tells you how you can prevent getting sick in the future besides washing your hands regularly.

Sickness is not just a problem for the physical self but a problem for all dimensions of self. Sickness affects us physically, mentally, emotionally and is caused when we fail to take appropriate steps toward real Wellness.

The current healthcare system is based solely on the idea of intervening when a sickness or disease has already occurred. But why not work towards preventive measures so that we never get sick? Sadly, much of the answer has to do with money. There is simply no profit in being well but there is profit in alleviating symptoms.

Did you think that you were doing all you could to stave off illness? You take your vitamins and drink your orange juice and get a nice amount of sleep. Do you tend to your spiritual needs? What about your mental or environmental needs? You cannot focus on only one aspect of Wellness and expect everything to be A-OK.

A negative amount of stress has a negative impact on your Wellness. If you overwork yourself but still take your vitamins, drink your juice, and sleep; you are still going to get sick. This is because you are failing to pay attention to your true Wellness. (This point cannot be said enough.)

Wellness is focused on preventive care. Unfortunately, many Americans live a fast-paced lifestyle that neglects our basic nutritional and Wellness needs and when we fall ill or develop a condition, we tend to lament, "Why me?!" The answer is that we need to rely on the current healthcare system to care for us when we need it but fail to think ahead and prevent disease and conditions before they happen.

The Destructive Power of Our Current Healthcare

But wait, you say, isn't the government doing all it can to bring about healthcare reform? We certainly hear about it every few years, but nothing ever seems to get resolved. We watch as politicians yell and stamp their feet that a change in healthcare is needed, necessary and far overdue. Sadly, while they may yell and scream until they are red in the face, things always seem to quiet down months later and the system has seen no real change.

All this noise does not change the fact that the current healthcare system is broken and has been for some time. As much as we may love our country, it's time to look at some basic facts: The healthcare system in the United States is just simply not the healthcare system that the American people deserve. The United States remains the only industrialized country that does not offer healthcare for everyone. Instead, we rely on complex insurance regulations and government agencies to provide help for those that need help or for those that can afford it, but that help is very rarely in the form of preventive care. The help that is offered is difficult to attain and often comes too late.

A majority of Americans are uninsured. Do you have insurance? If so you are one of the lucky ones. The masses of uninsured Americans go through life hoping that they don't get ill, that they don't develop anything devastating like cancer or heart disease, because they will be unable to pay for treatment—a goal that is admirable if they were also pursuing Wellness but they are not. They are simply crossing their fingers and hoping that Lady Luck will smile upon them.

If sickness does arise, the uninsured often wait until minor conditions become major before they rush to the emergency room, only to be hurried through the care process and given a huge bill at the end of services. And, they are still not truly well.

No one is telling us how to be well or how to truly take care of ourselves. Instead we are left to consume, ingest, devour and only think about our lifestyle when something bad happens. And when it does, we are sent to the hospital and doctors; hoping that they will have a magic pill to solve what ails us.

As a result, the average person is unable to ever be truly healthy. The average person must suffer not only the illness, but massive debt as well, accrued through medical treatments and interventions that could have been avoided altogether.

To illustrate just how harmful the current healthcare system is to the average person, let us look at some numbers. In this country there has been $77 billion in unnecessary costs, 20,000 deaths result every year from hospital errors, 12,000 of which from unnecessary surgeries and 7,000 deaths per year from medication errors. [2]

How many of these deaths could have been avoided if the system was focused on educating about Wellness and preventive care? It is hard to say, but certainly at least a handful of these deaths could have been prevented. A handful of families could have remained whole.

Profit, not the health and well-being of patients, has become the driving force in healthcare and we are suffering because of it. The current healthcare model is essentially destructive to the health of Americans.

This is not the fault of American citizens. This is a system that has been established for generations and one which is difficult to fight against. Luckily, for you, the American citizen looking for change, you are heading in the right direction. Through Wellness and preventive medicine, you will not only be able to take your own health and well-being in hand but you will also find a wellspring of opportunities waiting for you as well! So do not get discouraged or upset about the current state of things, because in order to make a change, you first need to know what to change.

This failure in healthcare results in unnecessary deaths and massive costs, which could be avoided if Wellness was the focus of the medical community. There is simply not enough profit in

---

[2]   Hoffman & Deitch, p. 5.

preventive care, as there is in treatment, for the companies that run the hospitals and for the big pharmaceutical companies.

In fact, the pharmaceutical companies are probably the largest contributor to the current healthcare crisis. Most of the research and development done by these companies focuses on the suppression of symptoms through drugs and pills. This thought process has permeated into our medical schools where the focus is on treatment of problems through surgery and disease management instead of actual care.

Instead, healthcare should focus on Wellness, the actualization of a healthy self in all dimensions and in all aspects of mind, body, and soul.

The True Cost of Healthcare

As a result of this perverse take on healthcare and how to properly care for those that need it, the United States is seeing the system collapse. At the head of this collapse is the continuing rise in the cost of healthcare.

The fact is that "the overall cost of healthcare doubled from 1993 to 2004"[3]. The cost of healthcare is expected to continue its rise in the coming years.

---

[3] Hoffman & Deitch, p. 3.

The skyrocketing healthcare costs are not the only obstacle that Americans must contend with. A faltering economy, a collapsed housing market, out of control debt, and a rising federal deficit is contributing to the inability for many families to pay for healthcare when they get sick.

This is leaving many Americans struggling to pay for basic healthcare and needs.

Employers are feeling the burden and many are reducing the amount of health insurance they offer employees. Health insurance is just too expensive for businesses to offer and far too expensive for individuals to purchase. Sure, there are programs like Medicaid and Medicare but many find these programs inaccessible since they either fail to qualify or still cannot afford the premiums.

What is attributing to the rising cost of healthcare, you may ask. Well there are several factors that attribute to the rise in cost.

New technologies and drugs contribute greatly to healthcare spending. New state of the art, innovative medical technologies are being developed each year. These technologies are costly and those costs need to be recouped by the manufacturers which mean that the consumers (patients) pay higher and higher fees and costs in order to have access to such technologies.

Prescription drugs to suppress and treat ailments and symptoms are growing ever costlier. The research and development of these drugs are passed on to consumers (patients) which increase healthcare spending across the board. Preventive care gained through an educated approach to Wellness would do wonders in reducing the need and demand for such drugs.

Chronic disease is driving up healthcare costs. Longer life spans and chronic diseases are placing a greater demand on drugs and treatments that are designed to only treat the physical manifestation of the disease. A lifetime of true Wellness, and not just focusing on the disease when it arises, could prevent much of the costs associated with chronic disease.

As a result, more than 15 percent of the United States's GDP is spent on medical care, 15 dollars out of every 100 dollars spent is "covering the cost of being sick". By contrast, universal health systems in other countries provide better care and are less costly: Canada: 8.4 percent of GDP, Sweden: 9.1 percent, Germany: 8.2 percent, Japan: 6.8 percent, United Kingdom: 6.2 percent. [4]

What is universal healthcare? Well, it's more than a simple campaign platform and buzzword.

Universal healthcare is where everyone, as long as they are a legal resident, is provided with basic healthcare. This means that the system is not based on who can pay, but rather the need of the individual. This is a radical idea, to say the least, and one that is observed in nearly every single country except the United States.

---

[4]   Hoffman & Deitch, p. 2.

But universal healthcare alone will not solve the out of control costs of healthcare in the United States. Preventive medicine and care must also be accessible for patients. The current system is simply not set up for preventive care. Universal healthcare encourages patients to seek help and treatment when problems first arise and not to wait until that small problem is a huge disaster.

The high cost of healthcare causes many to adopt a 'wait and see' attitude with their health. A nagging cough might go away. A shortness of breath, tightness in the chest might get better over time. Why then waste hundreds of dollars on tests and diagnosis? The result is a midnight run to the emergency room; a trip that could have been prevented if not for the out of control cost of healthcare. Universal healthcare provides these needed tests for individuals who would otherwise not be able to afford them.

To Keep Us Sick

The majority of funds spent on our modern healthcare system are simply unnecessary. In universal healthcare systems the focus is not on treating disease but on Wellness and disease prevention. In the United States we live with a disease based healthcare system where the focus is on treatment and not prevention.

A disease based healthcare system is designed to keep people sick. This is because American healthcare's major concern is not the health of her people but on the bottom line, the profit lining her pocket. Funding for new prescription medicines and new treatments are a top priority, so it is in the interest of a disease based healthcare system to keep people sick. If there were no sick people, who would fund all that research into the newest and latest drug?

Remember how much your last prescription was? It was pretty costly, I bet.

Universal healthcare is dependent upon a healthcare system that works in an opposite manner. This is why governments, such as the United Kingdom, spend so little on healthcare compared to the United States. Universal healthcare is focused more on Wellness and prevention or a Wellness based healthcare system. A Wellness based healthcare system then would cost less to implement than our current system.

What's more, a Wellness based healthcare system would include a far wider range of medicine and treatment. Healthy foods and alternative treatments will be considered viable treatment options under a Wellness based healthcare system.

A disease based healthcare system simply does not allow that yoga is a way to treat illness. Yoga is a way to prevent disease by helping to harmonize the Self. A disease based healthcare system allows for its participants to sit about the house, remain inactive and then treat the subsequent results of obesity and high blood pressure.

In fact, our current disease based healthcare system almost encourages us to sit about the house. Why? Because when we get ill, and we will, if all we do is sit on the couch, there are drugs and expensive surgeries that will let us avoid any negative consequences of our actions.

Lifestyle choice has everything to do with health. I will pause here and let you digest that statement. I know that statement is radical and really opposite to everything that you knew about health.

Poor lifestyle choices contribute to the majority of major diseases faced in this country. That is because people are simply failing to take good care of their health. We are responsible for ourselves and our lifestyle choices are a reflection of that.

The most common diseases, which are also the most costly, can be prevented in part or in full by smart habits and good lifestyle choices. These diseases are:

- Diabetes;
- Heart disease;
- Obesity; and
- Cancer.

Treating these diseases is expensive and can be deadly if left unchecked for too long. Our current disease based healthcare depends on people developing these ailments in order to continue operations. Spending money on treatment of these diseases is made necessary because the majority of the United

State population is ignorant of true Wellness and what lifestyle choices have to do with preventing disease and sickness.

Disease based healthcare is nothing more than a business, transforming doctors and other medical professionals into pencil pushing businessmen instead of caring physicians. By developing a system that focuses on Wellness, these doctors and professionals can go back to actually taking care of people instead of worrying about bottom lines and profit margins.

But this change is a radical one for many, especially for the healthcare industry which depends on treating those with heart disease, cancer, obesity, and diabetes and not educating people on prevention and Wellness.

Cardiovascular Disease

Cardiovascular disease is one of those conditions that can be avoided with proper preventive measures and appropriate lifestyle choices. The fact remains that cardiovascular disease causes 950,000 deaths a year in the United States.

Cardiovascular disease is any condition that affects the heart and blood vessels. One of the causes of cardiovascular disease is the build-up of fatty plaque.

There are several different forms of cardiovascular disease. Most of these forms can be prevented by proper diet and exercise. In other words the ability to make appropriate life style choice affects whether or not you might be diagnosed with cardiovascular disease.

Atherosclerosis is a build-up of plaque in your heart's arteries which causes arteries to harden, which restricts blood flow.

Atherosclerosis can be caused by:

- Obesity;
- Smoking;
- Poor diet; and
- Lack of exercise.

Heart arrhythmia is another type of heart disease which causes abnormal heart rhythms.

Causes of hearty arrhythmia can be:

- Smoking;
- High blood pressure;
- Diabetes;
- Use of alcohol and caffeine; and
- Stress.

Heart attacks are another form of this disease. Heart attacks can be attributed to:

- Poor diet;
- Stress;
- Smoking;
- Obesity; and
- Lack of exercise.

The point is that cardiovascular disease is one of the leading causes of death in America and is the leading cause of disability in working adults. But it does not have to be! A focus on Wellness and preventive care can greatly reduce the risk of developing this disease.

Not too many Americans are even aware that there is a way to reduce the risk of cardiovascular disease. Due to the disease based healthcare complex, we are not told about preventive measures to take. Why should we be? Cardiovascular disease costs Americans $400 billion a year in medical costs.

There are eight really simple steps that you can take to reduce the risk of cardiovascular disease. These preventive steps all fall in line with the idea of total Wellness of Self. They pay attention to all of the dimensions of Wellness and not just treating the physical manifestation of the disease when it happens. Why wait for a heart attack when you can work to prevent that trauma now? The answer is ignorance of what you can do and that ignorance is perpetuated by a healthcare system that has failed us all.

The eight steps you can take to help in the prevention of cardiovascular disease are:

1. Stop smoking: Smoking causes high blood pressure which increases the chances of heart disease and stroke. Smoking (and I do not mean to preach) is just an overall bad habit that contributes to bad health across the board. Even if you smoked all of your life, your risk of cardiovascular disease will decrease as soon as you quit smoking.

2. Controlling high cholesterol: High cholesterol can be prevented with the right diet. A diet that is low in cholesterol and saturated fat, but high in fiber, is best. You should also maintain a healthy weight through diet and exercise.

3. Controlling or preventing diabetes: Diabetes can greatly increase your chances of cardiovascular disease. Proper diet and exercise will go a long way in helping the prevention of diabetes and in turn of cardiovascular disease.

4. Controlling high blood pressure: While blood pressure medication is commonly used to treat people with this condition, proper life style choices can prevent the need of pills. Again, a proper diet and plenty of exercise are important.

5. Avoid excessive alcohol use: Alcohol, when used in excess, can be extremely detrimental to your health, not just your heart health but for your entire body. Alcohol increases your blood pressure which in turn increases your risk for heart attack.

6. Exercise: Really! I'm not sure how many times I can tell you how important adequate exercise is to Wellness.

7. Proper diet: Eat healthy foods, foods that your body craves, foods that do not come in a Styrofoam container.

8. Keep your weight at a healthy level: By keeping your Body Mass Index at an acceptable level, you will be preventing not only cardiovascular disease, but a host of other ailments.

Cancer

Everyone has been affected by cancer, either you have been diagnosed with it or you know someone who has. Cancer is one of the scariest diagnoses anyone can face. Over 1.3 million people are diagnosed with cancer each and every year. Of those 1.3 million, one third of cancer related deaths can be traced to poor lifestyle choices. This disease is a great focal point for debate on what causes it and how to treat it.

Today there are over 100 cancer related diseases recognized by the medical community. There are five broad categories that cancers can be grouped into. These categories are:

- Leukemia;
- Sarcoma;
- Carcinoma;
- Lymphoma; and
- Central nervous system cancers.

Cancer afflicts the cells. When a cell is damaged, it can mutate and over time these mutated cells join together to form a tumor. Tumors can either be benign or malignant. Benign tumors are not cancerous and be removed without fear of reoccurring. Malignant tumors, on the other hand, are cancerous and often spread to other areas of the body if left without treatment.

Often, people are unaware that they even have a tumor until the cancer has spread to several parts of their body. This is because the healthcare system is not set up to prevent cancer but to treat it once it has become a serious problem. High medical costs often prevent low income individuals and those without insurance to seek appropriate help, even if cancer has been detected.

Cancer counts for over $200 billion a year in health costs, yet many cancers can be prevented with a focus on proper Wellness. Cancer is not just a 'fact of life' and for many it is the result of poor choices.

Tobacco

Smoking, as I mentioned earlier, negatively affects all aspects of Self. True Wellness is a lifestyle without the use of tobacco of any kind. Tobacco use is not mandatory; you are not forced to smoke a pack a day. You choose to do it. You are making a poor lifestyle choice that can very well cause you to die an early death. Am I being overdramatic? I don't believe so.

Tobacco causes cancer of the:

- Mouth;
- Kidney;
- Esophagus;
- Larynx;
- Throat;
- Bladder;
- Cervix;
- Pancreas; and
- Stomach.

Physical Inactivity and Poor Diet

Poor diet and a lack of exercise greatly attributes to obesity. And, obesity has been shown to be the cause of several types of cancer, such as:

- Breast;
- Kidney;
- Endometrium;
- Colorectum; and
- Oesophagus.

Make sure to eat plenty of fruits and vegetables and limit that red meat intake. Having a good steak every once a while is a wonderful treat but certainly not a treat for every single night. Choose to eat a diet full of light and lean foods which will reduce the risk of obesity, thus reducing the risk of cancer.

Exercise regularly. Exercise is a terrific way of achieving Wellness. Aim for at least 30 minutes of vigorous exercise each day.

Cancer is a serious disease but many of the cancers can be prevented. Think back to your last trip to the beach. Did you wear sunscreen? Skin cancer can be prevented by simply being smart about the sun. Other types of cancer can be prevented in a similar manner, but using common sense and by practicing prevention.

By being focused on Wellness and not treatment, the risk of cancer can be greatly reduced.

Diabetes

Diabetes affects 18.2 million people with 798,000 new cases each year. Yet, diabetes can be prevented. Why then are there 200,000 deaths related to diabetes every year?

The answer is a healthcare system that is only focused on treatment and not prevention. The answer is a populace that is not properly educated on how to achieve adequate Wellness.

Diabetes is a metabolism disorder. When we eat, our body breaks the food down into a substance called glucose. The glucose enters our blood stream and our cells use it for energy. This process is possible thanks to a hormone called insulin, which our pancreas produces. In healthy individuals, the production of insulin happens automatically.

A person with diabetes is unable to produce insulin, or fails to produce enough insulin, and as a result has an increase of glucose in their blood stream. The cells are unable to absorb the glucose and do not receive the energy from it.

There are three types of diabetes. Type 1 is when you do not produce any insulin at all. Type 2 is when you fail to produce enough insulin. And, Gestational diabetes occurs only during pregnancy.

Failure to treat diabetes can result in a variety of diseases and ailments from hypoglycemia to cardiovascular disease. Once you are diagnosed with diabetes you have it for life. You must treat your diabetes with either insulin injections (for Type 1) or tablets (for Type 2) Both types of diabetes can benefit greatly from proper diet and exercise.

While there is currently no known way to fully prevent Type 1 diabetes, there are steps you can take to increases the odds in your favor. These preventive measures can also be used to help in the prevention of Type 2 diabetes.

Eating a proper diet: This is important, since a proper diet will help you keep glucose levels in check. If you are already diagnosed with diabetes, a healthy diet can go a long way in treating and managing the condition. There is a misconception that diabetic appropriate foods are bland and tasteless. A diet rich in fruits and vegetables as well as plenty of whole grains and legumes is essential.

SELVA SUGUNENDRAN

Adequate exercise: This will ensure that you keep your weight under control and in turn prevent diabetes. Thirty minutes of exercise a day is generally the agreed amount of time for many who suffer from diabetes.

Diabetes accounts for $100 billion in medical costs annually. Through prevention and proper management, for those already diagnosed with diabetes, you can reduce that amount drastically. America is a society that almost promotes diabetes. We live in a society of foods high in saturated fat where the word exercise is avoided like the plague.

Many American believe in fast and quick. When was the last time you stopped to think about the importance of exercising or how much fat is in a fast food burger? Don't feel bad if it has been a while. Now is the time to change. Wellness begins with a decision. That decision can be to prevent the onset of diabetes or the decision to better manage it.

Wellness and prevention can begin at any point of your life. You just have to take a step back from what you are used to and assess your lifestyle and behavior.

The Apple and the Donut

You wake to a screaming alarm clock and stumble into the kitchen for coffee and breakfast. On the counter are an apple and a donut. You know you should eat the apple. You know this.

It's the best choice. Apples are nutritious, healthy, and delicious. An apple a day keeps the doctor away, after all.

Donuts, however, are pretty tasty. Just look at that glaze! Donuts and coffee go hand and hand. How many times have you seen anyone dip apples in coffee? You know donuts have no nutritional value what-so-ever and that while donuts are delicious, they are certainly not healthy. Yet you are going to choose the donut each and every time. Why?

We are a people of instant gratification. As a society, the American people grossly undervalue the rewards that an apple will bring. Those rewards are not instantly realized and instead you must wait for those rewards. Donuts, on the other hand, are overvalued for the gratification they bring. That gratification is instantaneous and we fail to think far enough ahead to realize that what we perceive as a reward from eating the donut is actually going to be detrimental to our health. We call this the "apple—donut paradox".[5] This paradox demonstrates just how skewed our priorities are when it comes to health and Wellness.

For the most part, we know how to make healthy decisions. We know that the apple is far better than the donut. Yet many of us will still make the decision to eat the donut. You would never feed your dog pizza would you? Of course, not. Why? Because you know that pizza does not contain anything nutritious for

[5]   Chestnut, J. (2011). *The Wellness & Prevention Paradigm*. Victoria, BC: TWP Press, p. 79.

your dog. Your loyal Fido will gain absolutely nothing from eating that pizza except for a stomach ache.

Why then do you think that that same pizza will have any value for you? Pizza is not a vegetable. Why then do you insist replacing vegetables with a slice of pizza in your diet?

It is all about the ability to make appropriate lifestyle choices that will positively impact your Wellness. We consume foods that are high in saturated fat with more chemicals than what goes into making bubble wrap and wonder; "Why is my stomach so upset?", "Why am I always fatigued?", "Why do I have diabetes, or "Why am I overweight?"

You are not giving enough attention to all of the dimensions of true Wellness. You are constantly choosing the donut over the apple. And yes, the donut tastes good and the rewards instant but you are going to pay for it in the future and in possibly devastating ways.

Remember that Wellness has six dimensions and in order to achieve an actual healthy state you must take care that all these dimensions are in harmony. In order to do this, you must focus on making the right lifestyle choices even if they are hard to make, even if it means you forsake the donut for the apple.

A Proper Diet

How can you expect to feel good when you feed yourself bad food? Eating right is essential for proper Wellness. A proper diet promotes proper weight which, in turn, promotes Wellness and prevents disease.

Obesity is a leading cause of heart disease and diabetes and eating a healthy diet staves off obesity. Foods that are low in saturated fats and full of nutrients are ideal.

Below is a list of commonly healthy foods:

- Whole grains;
- Milk;
- Fruits and vegetables;
- Meats like poultry and fish;
- Legumes;
- Eggs; and
- Nuts.

You might look at this list and realize how obvious this is. Of course, whole grains are healthy and of course a diet full of fruits is the way to go, yet the majority of the population continues to choose the donut each time.

Adequate Exercise

There's that nasty little word again, exercise. It's not necessary to go to the gym or run five miles every morning before work. The kind of exercise I'm talking about is just enough to get your blood flowing and your heart pumping.

The more exercise the better, of course. Exercise is more than burning fat, it is about reducing stress, finding balance within yourself and achieving a new state of mind and body.

Yoga, jogging, weight lifting, really any kind of physical exercise contributes to Wellness.

You might have just realized that you knew all this. And that is the point. We already have the knowledge to live a healthy life and to make lifestyle choices that help us to achieve Wellness. This knowledge, in turn, helps us with preventive measures when it comes to our health.

The Choices We Live With

Despite knowing what is healthy and what makes for good lifestyle choices, many of us still insist on making poor decisions. We are conditioned to believe that our choices have no actual consequences, that we are able to do what we like and eat what we want and never have to face the results. This belief has helped to establish the current disease based healthcare system.

A woman who likes to eat nothing but tiramisu is going to get fat. Instead of exercising her way back to an acceptable weight, she is able to walk into a doctor's office and request a complex and expensive surgery that will rid her of all that unseemly weight. The reason for this is that we are trained not to think about the consequences of our actions. Why should we, when we have a healthcare industry that is built around treatment and not prevention.

Preventive care and Wellness begins when you take responsibility for your decisions. What you do now definitely matters later on. Remember the apple and the donut? Well, that donut tasted good but you will experience the benefit of the apple later on.

There is a marketing tactic called hyperbolic discount that helps to explain why we choose the instant gratification over the long term reward. We see healthy foods as having no real value, even though they do, because we cannot immediately experience the reward. So, the healthy food or healthy lifestyle choice is discounted in our view in favor of foods and a lifestyle that provides gratification instantly. Sounds complicated? Just think back to the apple and the donut paradox.

To you, it is just one donut. But that one donut soon adds up to a dozen, then two dozen and before you know it you are being diagnosed with diabetes. Or, you choose not to exercise for one day and then a week and soon you are obese.

If we fail to see the consequences of our actions immediately we simply do not think about for better or worse.

Marketing has a lot to do with this. Television and print ads often display poor lifestyle choices with happy, energetic, and beautiful people. That beer commercial is full of young happy adults enjoying a night out on the town. Those fast food ads show friends enjoying burgers with three patties and enough fries to fill a corn silo.

These ads fail to show that all that fast food is harmful to your health and too much alcohol increases your chances of developing heart disease.

The fact remains that as a society we must take responsibility for our actions. Wellness is about realizing that your actions directly impact your reality whether it is your health, your relationships, or even your career.

Since we cannot see our health decline immediately, from a life of drinking nothing but soda, we believe that we will not be affected. And since we cannot immediately see the benefits of drinking water, we fail to think about the positive impact it has on our bodies. If the result is not directly presented before us; we ignore it.

Instead we must think ahead and look forward.

Time For a Change

Our current thought process about lifestyle choices and Wellness must change. There is simply no excuse for it any longer. The fact is that "the vast majority of the people who are filling the hospitals, the vast majority of the people who are dying, are dying from suicide by lifestyle choice: they are dying from ignorance regarding the importance of lifestyle." [6]

---

[6]   Chestnut, p. 91.

There are five misconceptions about Wellness contributing to why people fail to make healthy lifestyle choices: availability, cost, confusion, time constraints, and taste concerns.

Availability

Good health is not something only the super-rich or affluent can afford yet proper health is touted as something that is expensive and hard to attain. The populace must be shown that Wellness is easily available to the masses.

In place of good decisions about lifestyle choices people are choosing things like fatty foods and believing that there is no alternative.

Cost

Fast food chains will have us believe that cooking at home, where we can enjoy a healthy meal with our loved ones, is far too expensive. Instead they offer a cheaper alternative with food that is high in saturated fat and encourages families to eat on the go rather than at the dinner table.

Confusion

Wellness, to the uninformed, is confusing. Wellness takes the concept of health that we are all familiar with and turns it on its head. Instead of focusing on only one part, physical, we must now look at other facets. What we once believed to be separate entities, the mind, body, and soul, are now connected.

Time Constraints

We are a busy people. We pack our schedules so full of errands and activities that we just do not have time to take adequate care of ourselves. This is simply untrue. Finding the time to do what matters is a part of Wellness. We are too stressed and too busy.

Taste Concerns

Healthy food tastes awful. This is the general consensus among many. Healthy foods are not bland pieces of cardboard. The excuse of not eating right because you do not like the taste is invalid.

Physically tasting items is not the only thing covered under taste concerns. You may find it unfashionable to exercise, or believe it is not in vogue to care about your stress but the result of that thought process is a lifetime of misery and poor health.

Those people rushing to the emergency room at 3:00 a.m. are buying into these five misconceptions about proper health. These are the people failing to take responsibility for their lifestyle and as a result are perpetuating the disease based healthcare system that dominates the United States.

This ignorance about what makes for a healthy individual is costing people their lives while lining the pockets of the companies that are supposed to be taking care of them. Education about proper Wellness is needed in order to move the country to a healthcare system where preventive care is the focus and where 3:00 a.m. emergency room visits are not necessary.

A change in behavior is also needed in order to move towards Wellness. Making the right lifestyle choices, to choose the apple over the donut as it were, may be difficult in the beginning but once you are committed to change; it will be easier with time.

Allowing people to continue killing themselves with poor lifestyle choices is wholly unethical on the part of policy makers and healthcare professionals. Change is desperately needed.

Conclusion

There exists in this country a dramatic disparity between healthcare and actual health. The current healthcare model of the United States is one built around the need to keep the population sick. It is the sick that pays the bills of insurance companies and companies whose primary focus is to make money in the healthcare industry.

This disease based healthcare system is based on treatment. The system is set up to treat the sick, to treat the injured, and to treat those facing possibly debilitating conditions—conditions which could otherwise be prevented, given the proper attitude about health and Wellness.

A preventive healthcare system is focused on keeping the population healthy. Such a system understands the needs of the Self and how important actual Wellness is.

A healthcare system that focuses on Wellness is also one that promotes smart lifestyle choices.

Lifestyle choices are important because our health is tied directly to the choices we make. If you choose not to exercise then that is your lifestyle choice and the consequence is going to be poor health. However, if you do choose to exercise, then you will be on your way to realizing the actualization of Wellness.

The United States is the only developed country that still focuses on helping people after they have gotten sick instead of educating the masses about preventive care. This allows the population to live under the assumption that no one is responsible for their actions. Pharmaceutical companies and the private corporations that own hospitals and healthcare facilities depend on the ignorance of consumers to keep their revenue up.

The American people are conditioned into accepting a lifestyle where they happily live in conditions that have been proven to be detrimental to their health. What's more, the majority of American people simply cannot afford adequate healthcare under the current system. Instead, they are forced to wait until a small symptom, like shortness of breath, becomes something devastating like a heart attack.

Other countries have a universal healthcare system where preventive care is the primary focus. In these countries people are able to seek out medical attention for that tightness of chest and receive the help needed to prevent a future heart attack.

Universal healthcare is more in line with the concept of Wellness and prevention. The primary concern of such symptoms is not to treat the disease but to prevent the disease in the first place.

The current disease based healthcare system in the United States is failing, to put it bluntly, and without reform the system will continue to fail until it completely collapses. There then exists a need in the country to create a healthcare system that is based on preventive care and not on treatment. Such a healthcare system is used to create Wellness for everyone.

By making proper lifestyle choices; eating right, and getting exercise; you can ensure that you will live a long and happy life. On the other hand, poor lifestyle choices will only lead to a life dependent on medication and expensive surgery.

Through education and reform we can establish a healthcare system that works in all facets of Wellness and not just in treating physical ailments when they happen. A healthcare system based on Wellness and prevention is the only way to ensure that everyone has access to the tools necessary for a healthy and happy life.

CHAPTER TWO

The Wellness Alternative: Preventative Healthcare

What is Preventive Medicine?

PREVENTIVE MEDICINE is crucial for a healthcare system that is focused, not on profit, but on actual health and Wellness. Wellness, as previously discussed, is the harmonizing of six individual dimensions of Self to promote and encourage true health.

Our current healthcare model fails to consider all six of these dimensions as a whole entity. Instead, the system focuses on only one at a time; this creates a healthcare system that is focused on treatments instead of prevention. Preventive medicine, on the other hand, understands that to achieve Wellness you must consider all six dimensions.

Preventive medicine and care focuses on the body, mind, and spirit as a whole entity. This belief, that care should be administered to all aspects of Self, is certainly not a new one. The practice of preventive care is one of the corner stones of

Eastern Medicine. Having balance in your life, and in your health, brings about a happier you.

It has only been in the recent decades that Wellness and preventive care has gained any kind of positive attention in the West. More and more people are becoming aware of just how important disease prevention is for their health and quality of life. When applied to the individual, preventive care focuses on proper exercise and a healthy diet as well as proper stress management.

Applied to the public, preventive care focuses on regulations about food safety, pest control, and vaccinations, all designed to help prevent diseases in the population. The basic idea behind universal healthcare, coincidentally, is the promotion of good health to the population. The belief is that if the population is healthy, through the proper upkeep of the environment, then the cost of healthcare can be greatly reduced.

In the United States, the only non-third world country that lacks universal healthcare, the current healthcare model is based not on prevention but on treatment. Medical professionals are just not paid to educate the public on preventive measures that they can take to stave off diseases and ailments. Instead, the American populace must first get sick before seeking any kind of medical attention. This creates unnecessary medical costs centered around the research, development, and creation of drugs and diagnostic tools that are all designed to treat rather than prevent.

It has been estimated that by 2013, the costs of prescription medication will be over $7 billion.[7] Why should millions of Americans pay this when the majority of their diseases and conditions could have been prevented through a Wellness program? It just makes no sense.

This runs in contradiction to the idea of Wellness. Wellness, based on keeping the Self healthy through the holistic approach to health by working on the six dimensions of Self (emotional, physical, social, environmental, spiritual, and mental), is the way to good health.

Preventive medicine and care understand the importance of these six dimensions and the need for individuals to keep these dimensions of Self in harmony. Disease based healthcare, the kind that the United States has, the kind that we are most familiar with, is simply unable to handle the need for preventive care. This is because the insurance agencies and other entities, that own and operate hospitals, do not find such practices profitable.

We can see this through the pharmaceutical companies. These companies make big bucks by developing pills and medicines used to treat and suppress symptoms instead of developing items that can be used to prevent or cure the disease.

Preventive care reduces the need for prescription drugs that are designed to only treat and suppress disease. As a result, prevention of disease is not widely practiced in the United State

---

[7]   Chestnut, p. 166.

since it reduces possible profit. However, several physicians and other professionals are now looking to the practice of preventive care and medicine as a viable solution of patient care. Preventive care, such as the kind found in universal healthcare systems, allows for doctors and physicians to actually care for patients instead of simply treating patients before sending them on their way.

Preventive medicine and preventive care has proven to be the best way of ensuring that the healthy stay healthy.

The Levels of Preventive Medicine

Preventive medicine has a variety of faucets and aspects that all work toward keeping you healthy. Being educated on these faucets and how they affect you and your health will go a long way in keeping you well.

When you are sick is no time to think about your health. You are already sick, after all and at this point the only thing you can do is treat the symptoms caused by the illness. Preventive care must begin when you are not sick, when you are perfectly fine and healthy and the very last thing you are thinking about is being sick.

Sure, there are going to be sacrifices but really anything worth doing is going to have sacrifices. A healthy lifestyle is one void of harmful substances and actions. Eating right, avoiding harmful habits like smoking, getting plenty of exercise, and getting enough sleep all go towards preventive care. Unlike our current healthcare model that works on the basis of treating those already sick and charging an obscene amount to do so, preventive healthcare works on the basis of avoiding illness altogether.

Keeping a healthy lifestyle and making good choices is the first defense against harmful conditions and ailments. Preventing such conditions and ailments negate the need for expensive medicine and treatment.

Finding health problems and diseases and then treating those conditions immediately is also considered preventive care. Uninsured Americans often wait for a condition to become serious before seeking medical condition. This is because basic healthcare is so expensive that for many, going to the doctor is just not economically feasible. They are then forced to seek medical attention when the condition becomes serious and can no longer be ignored.

While making healthy lifestyle choices can go a long way in preventing disease and harmful conditions, there are factors that cannot be changed such as genetics. It is important under a model of preventive care and Wellness to see a doctor for regular checkups. Again, the average American cannot afford what is considered among many a luxury expense. Many cancers can actually be cured if caught early. Other diseases can be treated early on to reduce the affects it has on your quality of life. It's all about prevention.

SELVA SUGUNENDRAN

However, this mindset of taking care of yourself before you get sick or before you get hurt is not practiced in the West. Instead, we rely on a system that treats us after the fact. As a result, we experience huge costs associated with healthcare making it impossible for the majority of Americans to afford adequate medical coverage. Whereas, preventive healthcare is an inexpensive alternative adopted by the rest of the world's industrialized nations.

Preventive medicine is not some unattainable goal and it is not some overly complicated industrial complex. It starts with you, how you live your life and the choices you make. Taking care of yourself now will result in a lifetime of good health. The main problem seems to be our attitude. We do not want to make an effort toward anything unless we see instantaneous results. This attitude must change in order to move toward a system based on prevention rather than treatment.

There are three levels of preventative medicine: Universal, Personal, and Specific. Each of these levels corresponds to a certain action or actions that should be done in order to follow the theory of preventive medicine. Remember that preventive medicine can be anything from brushing your teeth to seeking an annual colonoscopy. The goal is to take actions that reduce the chances of getting sick later on in life. While the rewards of choosing a healthy lifestyle will not be instantly noticeable, they do exist. You just have to develop a mindset of delayed gratification. While this might seem counter intuitive from everything our society stands for, it is really a much better alternative than serious illness and complications down the road.

Universal Preventive Care

The first level of preventive care is Universal and involves all aspects of society. This is also the level where common sense and reason reign. Most of us already know how to follow a preventive care plan based on the Universal level. Yet the majority of the population fails to follow a preventive care plan based on the ideals of this level.

This level is the most dependent upon proper lifestyle choices. These choices, eating right, avoiding addictive and harmful habits, and staying active are all things that everyone knows are healthy yet the majority of us simply fail to do them.

Basic preventative habits, like washing your hands to stop the spread of disease and getting plenty of exercise, are both things that everyone knows. These are preventive measures taken on a Universal level. No matter who you are or what you do, you can participate in these activities. Health is not the only focus at this level, since true Wellness does not begin and end with the physical body and physical ailments.

Remember, you must take care of yourself in all aspects of Wellness. Mental Wellness is just as important as physical Wellness. If you do your homework, for example, it will help to keep your mind sharp and allow you access to a wide range of educational opportunities.

Let us take a look at some aspects of Universal preventive care individually in an effort to gain a better understanding of the concept. As mentioned before, this level of preventive care involves society as a whole from schools to businesses and includes the individual.

A proper diet is not about depriving yourself of tasty food and it is not about achieving a size 0. A proper diet is about eating foods that your body needs, food that give you energy and make you feel great. A proper diet can reduce your risks of heart disease, cancer, and even depression.

Not too many of us give much thought to what we eat. We are a nation of fast food junkies, so to make a lifestyle change that is essential for life, you will have to start slow. Make gradual changes to your diet that meets your body's nutritional demands. You do not have to have rice cakes for dinner but substituting fruit for a chocolate bar or some healthy yogurt for an ice-cream cone, means that you are on your way to a proper diet.

Wellness and preventive care is more than just watching what you eat. It is about proper stress management and developing proper skills to cope with everyday life. Exercise, volunteer work, even reading for enjoyment are all part of the concept of Universal Wellness.

The idea of this level of preventive care is to focus on the most basic prevention situations. And most of it is advice that we have all been told since childhood. Take your vitamins, say your prayers, do your homework, don't smoke, don't drink, and wash your hands after you use the bathroom are what we tell children and that advice is preventive medicine.

As adults, preventive care advice is a bit different though we should still listen to the advice we were given as children. Going in for check-ups and screenings of common conditions and disease is a must. Continue to brush your teeth, walk in the evening, and attend educational classes on topics you enjoy.

Preventive care focuses on what makes you happy, because if you're happy then chances are you are on your way to being healthy as well. Universal preventive care is what everyone no matter gender, race, genetic disposition, or economic status needs to do in order to achieve Wellness.

Personal Preventive Care

Often, the need for preventive care is right before our eyes. Personal preventive care is the act of taking responsibility for the diseases and conditions that we know we may be predisposed to. In these instances the need for prevention and the type of preventive medicine we need is obvious, yet many choose to ignore it.

The whole idea of preventive care is to take action when it comes to your health before major complications arise. If you knew that in the future you were going to get heart disease, why would you refuse to do anything about it until it's too late? This just does not make sense, yet this is what the majority of the population does; they wait. Thanks in large part to our disease based healthcare system, we've been conditioned into believing that when it comes to diseases, there is not much we can do until the disease manifests. Only then can we seek any type of medical attention, usually in the form of expensive prescription drugs or costly treatments.

If you know that there exists in your family a history of diabetes or heart disease or any medical condition, you need to be vigilant against such conditions. This means making an effort toward your best health. The earlier you start preventive care, such as eating right or exercise, the better your chances are at avoiding disease altogether or at the very least minimize the extent and seriousness of it.

On a social level this type of preventive care can be used to distinguish at-risk groups and target health campaigns for them. The anti-drug rhetoric is just such an example, mostly targeted toward teens in urban areas, the anti-drug campaign attempts to prevent future drug abuse. This is a form of personal preventive care as it targets a condition; drug abuse, and the group of people likely to experience the condition; teens.

Preventive care is essential to reach a balanced state of Wellness. While a disease based healthcare system fails to properly promote preventive medicine, because if they did how would they earn as much profit as they do now? Until the healthcare system undergoes reform, we must be proactive when it comes to preventive care. Ultimately we are responsible for ourselves. While we would like to believe that we can shirk responsibility, there comes a point when such behavior comes back to us. Eventually, we all must face the consequences for the life we choose to lead.

If you ignore your family history of diabetes and continue to live a lifestyle of poor dietary choices without any physical activity; you will, in almost all certainty, develop diabetes. However, if you maintain a proper diet and get plenty of exercise; you just may avoid diabetes all together. Preventive medicine on this level is important in determining how healthy you are going to be in the future.

The major obstacle here is that we hate to delay gratification and that is what has to be done on this level of preventive care. If you know that you have a higher than average likelihood of developing a condition than your peers, then you must follow a stricter diet or you have to abstain from pleasures like drinking or smoking cigarettes.

As a society, if we see that a portion of the population is more predisposed to harmful behavior such as drug abuse or even obesity, then we must take preventive care actions. Measures like education and ad campaigns espousing the dangers of drugs and the negative impact of greasy fried food is a way of doing just this.

The bottom line is that you have got to take responsibility for yourself and your actions, at an early age, in order to avoid complications further down the line.

Specific Preventive Care

Specific preventive care is taking care of issues and complications, as they arise, before they impact the quality of your life in an extreme way. The goal is to prevent a condition from worsening. Usually this is the stage where most of us seek medical attention, but ideally you should work toward a state where this stage is unnecessary.

Now, there are instances where this is impossible. Genetic disorders, unforeseen accidents, and similar situations are hard to fully control, let alone predict. In these cases, targeting the specific conditions and then working on preventing them from worsening is the goal.

This is also the case if you begin focusing on Wellness at a point in your life after you are diagnosed with a condition. Managing diabetes is important to ensure that you have a good quality of life. Knowing that such a condition exists and then how to properly manage that condition, through insulin injections, proper diet, and exercise is a form of specific preventive care.

For the most part, when we talk about specific preventive care, the idea is to avoid traditional medical intervention. For example, if you notice that you are packing on a little extra weight and are now bordering on an unhealthy weight; you are going to want to work on loosing that weight. If you just allow yourself to continue gaining weight, you are going to become obese. And obesity can then lead to heart disease, high blood pressure, and any other host of serious complications associated with weight gain.

Medical conditions are not the only topic that this preventive medicine area covers. Preventive medicine and Wellness plays a part in all areas of our lives. It is important to understand that a balance of Self must be struck in order to achieve true health. Teachers and parents who notice a student's performance begin to slip, might want to take action immediately. Waiting may result in that student failing a crucial class or completely failing a grade. Falling grades can even be an indicator of something far more serious than not understanding a particular chapter.

Falling grades can be a symptom of a far more serious issue. Drug use is one such explanation, as is trouble at home, or even a condition such as ADHD. By working under the theory of specific preventive care teachers, parents, and guidance counselors should take steps to curtail this symptom and work to correct it.

Social ailments too can benefit from this type of preventive care. It is hard to notice when you start to isolate yourself from friends and family. It happens to almost everyone at some point in our lives. Whether it is due being over worked, feeling stressed, or even feeling a little blue, at some point we all alienate ourselves from peers and loved ones. This behavior, if left unchecked, can have devastating effects on Wellness.

It is important to have meaningful interactions with others. If you do not care to spend time with peers, then volunteer your time at a children's hospital or other similar cause. Humans need other humans. If you see a friend alienating him or herself, then force them to interact with you or at least with someone else.

Wellness can only be achieved if you are willing to make an effort to work toward it. The three levels of Wellness; Universal, Personal, and Specific are designed to help you determine what type of preventive care you may need for nearly any given situation. While some of these situations will overlap, the primary factor to remember is prevention.

You must work toward keeping yourself healthy, not after you fall ill, but before you even get the sniffles.

Habits Are Hard to Break Even the Bad Ones!

Changing your lifestyle is no easy task. It takes a tremendous amount of willpower and strength, both qualities that we all possess. It is up to you then to implement change. There are three ways to change bad habits; whether it be chewing your nails or living a lifestyle counterproductive to Wellness.

It is first important to make the decision. Say it out loud. "I am going to work toward Wellness," or however you would like to state your decision in your own words. Secondly, you are going to ignore the feeling that something is not right. It may not "feel right" to get up and take a walk every morning or to drink more water instead of a soda. You may think that you are not acting like yourself. But you are just a healthier version of you. And last, you are going to want to work toward this change each and every day. Do not take a day off and give yourself a break. Do not justify missing a day of walking because you just do not feel up to it. You have to push yourself in order to reach your goal.[8]

Wellness Plan

A Wellness Plan is an important tool in the journey to Wellness. A proper plan will act as your road map, guiding you and aiding you to those important lifestyle choices that are so crucial in preventing disease and staving off harmful conditions and circumstances.

A proper Wellness Plan is one that is customized for you. The plan should address your own unique needs and circumstances. You cannot simply go online and follow a Wellness Plan that was designed for someone else, since it will not have your own

---

[8]   Hoffman & Deitch, p. 295.

needs in mind. That plan might be for a champion boxer and not for an over stressed soccer mom.

The Wellness Plan is all about taking charge of your own life and of the circumstances that dictate your life. The Wellness Plan is designed to help you in the prevention of harmful and negative factors that affect your life.

A proper Wellness plan will take into consideration the six dimensions of Wellness.

We can break the Wellness Plan into three categories: Daily, Weekly, and Monthly. Each category will address what you can and should do to ensure continued Wellness.

Remember, the path to Wellness is not an easy one, it takes time and dedication, but once achieved, the benefit will far outweigh any difficulty you faced along the way.

Daily Plan

- Sleep: The importance of sleep cannot be overlooked. Getting enough sleep is crucial to maintain your mental and physical health. While everyone has their own requirements for the amount of sleep they need, it is important that you actually get plenty of sleep and a good quality sleep at that.

- Calm: We lead stressful lives. Sometimes stress is beneficial but too much stress can be detrimental to our well-being. Finding time to relax and to reflect is important to maintain Wellness. You might think that you just do not have the time to go off on your own to relax, but you will need to make the time. You don't have to sit and mediate. You can paint, read, or take a long aimless walk, as long as it gives you time to reflect and relax. Aim for 5 to 20 minutes of quiet reflection.

- Exercise: It isn't necessary to hit the gym but as long as you get off the couch and move, move, move! Thirty minutes of daily exercise is necessary to keep your heart, lungs, and mind healthy and active.

- Eating Well: Remember to avoid too much food that is high in saturated fats. Eat fruits, vegetables, whole grains, and other foods that will provide fuel for your body, mind, and spirit.

Weekly Plan

- Find a Hobby You Enjoy: Participating in an activity that you enjoy, whether it's crocheting, model building, or scrap booking—participating in a hobby keeps your mind sharp. And, it never hurts to have a little fun.

- Meet With Friends: Our social and emotional health is just as important as our physical or mental health. Humans are social animals; we thrive on interacting with others. Meeting for coffee, talking on the phone and just spending time with someone we enjoy, goes a long way in achieving true Wellness.

- Heavy Activity: This just means participating in an activity that puts a bit more strain on you than simply walking around the block. Participating in the company softball league or bowling league is a good example. Hiking every weekend is another example.

Monthly Plan

Once every month take yourself somewhere special. Treat yourself to dinner or a movie or spend some time at a spa or have a massage. Plan to do whatever it is you enjoy and you are contributing to your Wellness.

A Wellness Plan is a very personal thing. Customize your plan to fit your life and lifestyle. Start small and make your goals attainable so you avoid any frustration. Even a minor change toward Wellness is a good thing.

Remember, your Wellness Plan needs to focus on all areas of your life. Take time to exercise, find some time for quiet reflection, eat right, help others, learn something new, and interact with people. All these things should be part of your Wellness Plan.

Wellness and Leisure Time

Preventive medicine and care is a lifestyle. When you decide to work toward a holistic approach to health, you are adopting the idea of preventive healthcare. This means that you are dedicating time and energy to methods of preventing illness and other negative influences that will have a harmful impact on your health.

As part of that dedication to lifestyle change, you are going to have to alter behavior that you were once used to and this means activities you enjoy during your down time as well.

Many of us spend our leisure time lounging about the house watching television or surfing the internet. Such activities have their time and place but many of us do nothing but just sit around. This is counter intuitive to Wellness. Living a sedentary lifestyle will only promote conditions such as heart disease and even depression. The human body was designed to move. It makes no sense to sit on the couch for twelve hours at a time, justifying such actions by saying it is our day off and this is how we spend our leisure time.

Instead, spend that leisure time doing something that will actually be beneficial to your mind, body, and spirit. You might be wary of making such extreme changes all at once, that is understandable. Strive to do at least one other activity, other than sitting on a couch, during your day off. It can be something like taking a walk around the block, preparing lunch for friends, or reading a book. Just as long as the activity you choose is a step toward your health and Wellness.

Really, there cannot possibly be anything so important and interesting on television for which you are willing to sacrifice your health. Instead of watching television, get up and get out of the house. Other possible activities can include:

- Hiking;
- Swimming;
- Painting; and
- Crafts.

As long as you are up and moving, even a little, you are still moving toward good health. Let's take a quick gander at some of the benefits of walking. You may think that a walk around the block could do little in making you healthy but walking has been shown to help prevent heart disease, stroke, and can even reduce the risk of breast cancer.[9]

Just because your day off is called leisure time does not mean you have to spend it doing nothing. Sure, the rest of your time is busy running errands, working hard, and taking care of others and you are entitled to some leisure time and do with it what you will. However, you must change your attitude about health and Wellness in order to redefine what leisure time means to you.

Just as with other faucets of your life; leisure time should be used to work toward the development of healthy attitudes and activities. In fact, leisure time presents possibly the best opportunity for focusing on your Wellness, since you normally have nothing else that is going to demand your attention during that time.

Relaxing and taking time out for yourself is a necessary part of Wellness but it is easy to overdo it. You are going to have to make the conscious decision to turn off the TV. If you do need to sit and relax, you can do it with a book or crossword puzzle—something that exercises your mind.

Your leisure time can be spent doing volunteer work, offering your time helping others and making a difference in the community is important to your overall Wellness.

---

[9]   Chestnut, p. 185.

The key is to redefine your leisure time to focus on prevention of illness. It is so easy to spend any down time sitting around, eating junk food and watching TV. Wellness encompasses all aspects of your life from the time you wake up to the time you go to sleep.

Wellness in the Workplace

The majority of Americans are employed. Many of those employed have positions that do not promote any kind of physical activity. Most of the jobs today are sedentary involving sitting behind a computer with fingers curled over a laptop. It is really no wonder why there are correlations being drawn between sedentary workplace and obesity in America.

It is hard to avoid weight gain when 8 to 12 hours of your day is spent sitting down. Such a sedentary lifestyle fails to promote healthy eating and really any positive impact upon your Wellness. This lack of focus on Wellness in the workplace is beginning to take its toll and not just on your silhouette, but on the employer's bottom line as well.

A recent movement in healthcare has employers thinking more seriously about Wellness in the workplace. These employers are beginning to understand that Wellness and healthy lifestyle choices have an impact on the way they run their business.

Unhealthy employees, who suffer from heart disease or diabetes, cost their company money. This is because an overall employee productivity decline when the workplace is unwell not only is the case but health cost skyrockets due to medical expenses and insurance coverage. As a result, some employers are beginning to adopt a preventive medicine philosophy in the work place. It has been shown that, "Workplace Wellness program(s) saved 33.6 percent on per person healthcare costs, reduced sick leave by 22.2 percent". [10]

Employers are beginning to take notice of harmful factors such as stress in the workplace and how it impacts their employees. To combat stress, many employers are implementing stress reducing activities in the office. These activities are designed to allow employees the chance to step away from their desk and take just a few minutes to relax. Massage, breaks, and other stress reducing activities are beginning to appear in more and more offices.

Employers are even introducing physical activity into the workplace. Some companies are welcoming yoga instructors into the office a few times during the work week. This allows employees time to exercise, breathe, step away from their high stress occupations and enjoy an activity designed to bring about optimal Wellness.

---

[10]   Chestnut, p. 185.

~78~   SELVA SUGUNENDRAN

Some companies are even offering incentives for employees who enter into programs that are designed to help people stop smoking. This new focus on preventive care means that bad habits like smoking should be done away with. Smoking leads to diseases that can be prevented if that person simply did not smoke.

Workplace Wellness is being taken seriously by employers who are hoping to improve employee efficiency. Workplace Wellness should be adopted because being healthy means that you are happier. Wellness is important in all areas of one's life from work to areas of your personal life. By developing a well-rounded and balanced life, where Wellness and health are the focus, and preventive measures taken to ward off the possibility of sickness and physical ailments, then both employees and employers can truly reap the rewards.

You should not sit back and wait for your company to adopt the Wellness attitude in your workplace. Now is the time to take action. Bike to work, get enough sleep, sit up straight—these are just some of the improvements you can make today.

It is important to get at least 30 minutes of aerobic activity every day. The purpose of aerobic activity and exercise is to get your heart pumping. This strengthens your heart, reducing the risk for a variety of diseases and even stroke.[11]

---

[11] Chestnut, p. 89.

Spiritual Wellness

Wellness, as you know by now, has six dimensions. Each of these dimensions needs to work in harmony in order to achieve a healthy and happy life. Wellness is the holistic approach to health and is achieved through preventive care and smart lifestyle choices.

One of the dimensions of Wellness, the Spiritual, is little discussed in today's Western society. In the case of Wellness, spirituality is not talking about religion or a belief or disbelief of God. Spiritual Wellness is when you achieve a state of existence where you are at peace with yourself and your surroundings. Holy men from around the Globe have been trying to achieve deep spiritual Wellness for centuries. All you are required to do is to reach a level of spiritual Wellness that promotes health and Wellness. If you choose to pursue it further, that is up to you.

Developing a healthy spiritual Wellness is not going to happen overnight. It is a deeply profound introspective journey. Being aware that you should work on your spiritual Wellness is a good first step on the journey.

First you will want to ask youself, 'Who am I?' 'Why is there evil?' 'Why do we (humans) exist?' These questions will get your thought processes flowing. Many great thinkers throughout history have tried to answer these questions and many of their answers are in direct conflict with their peers. So don't feel bad if the answers you come up with are not the same as what others think.

Part of spiritual Wellness is being tolerant of others' beliefs and opinions. This acceptance allows us to see the people and not just their belief systems or the stereotypes we attach to them. Acceptance also allows us to live a life free from placing blame on others. We are the ones that make mistakes and we should be able to step up and accept that.

Make a connection with the inner you through art. Music, dance, painting, and any other form of artistic endeavors put us in touch with our Self. When we are in tune with our Self, we are in tune with our Wellness. Art also allows us to grow through the pursuit of knowledge and curiosity.

Find a time to get away and be quiet. We surround ourselves with noise. Noise from the TV, the chatter of the radio, the roar of traffic—all this noise bombards us every single day. This causes terrible stress. Find time to enjoy the quiet. Meditation is a good way to do this. Sit in a quiet room, close your eyes, and breathe deeply. Just enjoy the silence. Enjoy the state of being.

Spiritual Wellness encompasses many aspects of our lives. You do not necessarily have to prescribe to any religion to find spiritual Wellness. All you have to do is be willing to ask deep and profound questions. Do not be afraid of looking for the deeper meaning in life. Life can be a wonderful and scary experience. Our spirituality is what allows us to explore and understand life.

Wellness Goals

In order to achieve total Wellness, it will be important to assess your current Wellness state and set specific goals to achieve it. Remember, achieving true Wellness is more than just eating more fruit or taking a walk around the block, it is really about making lifestyle changes.

You are going to change your attitude and how you go about living your everyday life. The changes you make are going to be small to begin with. A change in habit here, a change in habit there, but as time goes on you will be able to add more changes until you are living a fulfilled life dedicated on your personal Wellness.

Before you jump into the task of changing your life, first take time to make a personal assessment of your health and Wellness. This assessment will serve to illustrate which areas of your life need improvement. The assessment will not only focus on your physical health, but in areas such as your social, mental, and spiritual needs. Wellness encompasses all areas of your life.

By making a proper assessment of your life and lifestyle you will be better able to determine which preventive medicine and care is best for your situation. It is important to develop a personalized Wellness assessment so the goals that you set will have an actual impact. A Wellness assessment comprises of two parts: family medical history and lifestyle.

Your family medical history is going to give you an idea of complications, conditions, and diseases that you may be susceptible to. By learning about the health issues faced by family members you will be better able to determine your level of risk and what steps and preventive measures you should be taking in an effort to avoid such complications.

Ask family members if diabetes, heart disease, and alcoholism or addictive behavior runs in the family. This will give you an idea of what areas of your life to change. If your family has a history of alcoholism, then cut back on the drinking. If Grandpa Jack had Type II diabetes, then work on adopting a healthier diet. Preventive medicine is designed to curtail any possible illness or ailments early on and not to treat them when they arise. Be proactive about your health.

Lifestyle choices play an important role in your health and Wellness. By assessing the choices you make, you will then be able to see what changes can be made in the name of better health.

Ask yourself questions about your lifestyle choices and daily habits and see how they scale. You will want good lifestyle choices to happen more often than poor lifestyle choices.

Below are some questions, divided into the six dimensions of Wellness, that you can ask yourself:

Physical

- Do I maintain a healthy weight?
- Do I exercise every day?
- Do I get enough sleep?

Social

- Am I honest and open with people?
- Do I engage in social activities?
- Do I strive to be a better person?

Emotional

- Do I deal with anger in a responsible way?
- Am I stable and well-adjusted?
- Do I feel good about myself?

Environmental

- Do I keep my surroundings neat and tidy?
- Do I spend enough time outside?
- Do I care about the environment?

Spiritual

- Do I believe that life is precious?
- Do I care for others around me?
- Do I work to create a life of peace and balance?

Mental

- Am I ruled by my emotions?
- Do I learn from my mistakes?
- Do I engage in learning for the sake of learning?

Of course there are other questions that could be asked in the sake of Wellness but these are just an example.

Once you realize where your current state of Wellness stands, you can then decide on a series of goals that will be designed to improve your overall Wellness. The key here is to start small. You are changing your lifestyle, by deciding on how you live your life, what decisions you make and the habits you keep.

Say that you do not keep a clean work area. One of your goals can be to tidy the area and organize any clutter or paperwork. Eventually the goals you set and achieve will move you toward Wellness. In a month's time take a look at the dimensions of Wellness again and compare how your new answers compare to the old.

The Improvements of Wellness

Perhaps the most noticeable reward you will see as you work toward Wellness and true health will be feeling good. This is the most important Wellness improvement. You will feel good, simply good. How many times in our lives of fast food and lethargy can we ever say that we feel good? Not very often I would bet.

By making lifestyle changes and working toward bringing balance to all dimensions of Wellness, you will notice that your attitude will improve, that you will no longer feel weighed down by physical and emotional burdens, you will better be able to interact with others and you will have a positive outlook on life.

You cannot put a price tag on feeling good so let's look at some other improvements that have quantitative values. Insurance costs will decline as a result of achieving a better state of Wellness. By showing insurance agencies that you are reducing your risk of cancer, heart disease, and other common ailments; you may be given a reduction on insurance premiums.

Of course, you will find that you are actually saving money on your way to Wellness. Cooking healthy means options at home rather than going to fast food joints, which will save some cash. While fast food is quicker and easier, it is also expensive and unhealthy.

Walking or bicycling instead of driving up the street, in an effort to improve your health, will save you a nice bit of gas money. Gas is not cheap and, let's face it, many of us simply cannot afford to feed our car gas every single day. Walking or biking is a great way to improve health and save some money.

Working towards Wellness will save you money on healthcare costs, reducing your need to keep lofty insurance premiums and can even eliminate the need for certain prescription drugs. Wellness will also save you money in your day to day life as well.

It has been estimated that the average 30 year old in America who adapts a wellness plan successfully and stays well could theoretically save upwards of $1 million if he or she lives up to 65 years.[12] This is a significant amount of money that can be better spent on other items and services. If you think about this, money can be put back into the Wellness market to help maintain a consumer's current state and even to improve upon it.

The most important improvement is feeling better about yourself in all areas of life. Not only will you be healthier physically but emotionally, mentally, and spiritually as well. You will find that you are better able to relate to those around you and you will feel more connection in your family and in your community.

Wellness and National Policy

The benefits of preventive healthcare and Wellness is taking center stage in the current healthcare debate. Politicians and

---

[12]   Hoffman & Deitch, p. 344.

presidential candidates often touch upon preventive care as a way to rally support for their cause. For the millions of Americans who are sick of the current disease based healthcare system, preventive care and Wellness is not just a hot button political topic, it is a way to true health and Wellness.

The current administration has taken preventive healthcare policy to the next stage and is attempting to make it national policy, much to the chagrin of staunch conservatives who may be benefiting from the current system of treatment. On the administration's side are facts and figures supporting that prevention, and not a system based only on treatment, will save Americans much needed money. Wellness is the idea of avoiding potentially life threatening diseases and complications through a holistic approach. This prevention means that Americans must actively participate in their own health, instead of waiting for conditions to get bad enough before seeking medical attention.

Living a life of Wellness creates a happier and healthier population. We can all benefit from a preventive healthcare system yet there are politicians and agencies who are actively working against new policies that promise a renewed focus on prevention of disease.

The National Prevention, Health Promotion and Public Health Council was created to provide an opportunity for Americans to participate in a healthcare system based on prevention. This council understands the importance of education and Wellness and encourages everyone from the individual to billion dollar corporations to participate. The ultimate aim is to bring affordable preventive care to all Americans.

In 2010, First Lady, Michelle Obama, created the Let's Move! campaign. The campaign's goal is to tackle childhood obesity and to educate the population about the importance of Wellness. Eating right and exercising are two important parts of this campaign but it is hoped that the children taking part in Let's Move! will grow up to live a life of prevention.

Along with Let's Move! is the creation of the National Prevention Strategy. The goal of this program is to create a nation of Wellness and health. By promoting preventive medicine and healthy lifestyle alternatives, the program is designed to revolutionize the current healthcare model.

The National Prevention Strategy focuses on seven priorities. These are:

- Preventing alcohol and drug abuse;
- Promoting a tobacco free lifestyle;
- Eating healthy;
- Sexual health;
- Mental and Emotional Wellness;
- An Active lifestyle; and
- A life free of violence.

As the importance of preventive medicine gains popularity for policy makers, we are certain to see more and more programs designed to promote ultimate Wellness.

Wellness is not just another diet trend or self-help guide, it is a lifestyle that has real, measurable results.

Conclusion

Wellness is not some craze that will simply disappear at the turn of next season. We are at a breaking point with our current disease based healthcare system. People are crying for a change and that change is a movement towards preventive care and Wellness. Knowing this you can optimize your opportunity for personal profit by assessing which aspect of Wellness can be utilized to earn the most money.

Preventive care is of great interest to baby boomers who are depending more and more on our current disease based healthcare to provide treatment for preventable diseases. And for Generation X'ers, the members of Generation X are going to continue looking at preventive care as a way to avoid the medical hardships experienced by their parents, which presents fantastic opportunities for the savvy businessperson.

You have the advantage because you can see where the market trends are moving. Wellness and preventive care is going to be a lucrative business and to ignore it is ridiculous. Begin now to determine how to get in on the ground floor of the Wellness campaign by analyzing the market, realizing where the most potential profits lie, and how to get to it.

CHAPTER THREE

Wellness for Profit

S O FAR ON our journey we have explored the current failing of the disease based healthcare industry and how Wellness and preventive care is the answer to what ails us. The Wellness industry promises to deliver fantastic results, not just in revolutionizing how we view health, but for those with enough foresight to take advantage of this burgeoning market.

Truly, the current system of healthcare is simply not destined to last much longer. As more and more consumers and patients are realizing that the true answer to health lies not in a treatment or sickness based system, but in a preventive care system, they will begin to look for a viable alternative. That alternative is Wellness.

Many attribute this growing interest in Wellness to the Baby Boomers, those children of post-World War II, that have for decades dictated much in the economy. As Baby Boomers are aging they are beginning to take special note of their health and are trying to find a way to stay young, vibrant, and energetic. For these Baby Boomers, Wellness is the answer. And, as they have done with so many other products and services, Baby Boomers have led the nation, and indeed the world, in a new way of thinking about health and healthcare.

With this new interest in Wellness and preventive care, entrepreneurs, business men and women, and in fact anyone with drive and motivation, are beginning to take advantage of this new market. The benefits of entering into the business of Wellness are of two-fold. By helping to spread the idea of Wellness, you will be helping many consumers who are sick and tired of the current way medicine works and second, you will be making a nice profit in the process. Who can ignore such a great opportunity?

The Next Big Thing

Calling Wellness the 'next big thing' is really not doing it justice. Remember that Wellness is a whole new way of thinking about the body, mind and spirit and how those elements correspond to health. Wellness is a multi-dimensional entity and if you ignore one or more of these dimensions, you are ignoring your potential for a happy and truly healthy individual. In fact, you are only taking advantage of a fraction of your potential if you fail to take proper care of your Wellness.

Wellness is a concept that affects and influences every single aspect of our day to day lives. Wellness is a lifestyle. By adapting to this lifestyle, you will be committing yourself to living in new and different ways than you were once so accustomed to. No longer will you be able to hop down the street and grab a greasy burger. Instead, you will have to weigh that burger carefully against your other choices; healthier choices. Of course, the results of such a lifestyle change will quickly make themselves known through increased energy, lost weight, and an overall feeling of well-being.

If you continue to choose poor lifestyle choices, such as the pesky donut over the delicious apple, then you will also see the results of that through fatigue, obesity, and continued sickness.

Patients, consumers, Baby Boomers, members of Generation X, and anyone with an idea of what being healthy might mean, are beginning to realize that Wellness is the only path to health. Wellness and preventive care works almost in direct opposition to the current disease based healthcare system that relies on consumers to get sick before doing anything about it.

It is beginning to make much more sense to many to prevent getting sick in the first place, instead of seeking treatment after the fact. This is opening up a whole new area of business; one that is focused on providing preventive care and medicine.

Wellness: More than a Trend

Wellness is far more than a trend, it is a lifestyle change. This change must depend on a new industry and market to support it. At the birth of Wellness decades ago, subscribers were hard pressed to find a place to buy healthy alternatives to overly processed food, or day to day products like soap, shampoo, or even exercise equipment.

Now, as Wellness is beginning to take center stage, more and more store fronts, businesses, and even food establishments are appearing that cater to those who have decided to pursue this lifestyle change. This in no way means that the market is full and there's no more room; in fact the Wellness Industry is just taking off, which means that there are plenty of opportunities for those that are prepared to take advantage of it.

Wellness has five characteristics that will ensure its continued survival.

Affordability

While at the start of the Wellness movement, products and services were not readily available or affordable—this is different in today's market place. This is in thanks to new technology and manufacturing capabilities that create products more efficiently. As demand continues to increase for these products and services, the prices will continue to decline. This worked much in the same way that new entertainment products exploded onto the market at astronomical prices only to drop within the year to become much more affordable.

Wellness products and services are now generally affordable for the masses, including low income families and individuals.

SELVA SUGUNENDRAN

This is due in part to massive retail giants and even popular restaurants offering healthier alternatives to what was traditionally fatty or loaded with sugar.

Legs

This simply means what the chances good for the Wellness product or service to move off the shelf on its own, long after all the advertisements and promotions leave the common market place. Wellness is a much desired state of being that is not so easily packaged and once all television ads stop airing, it will not simply vanish from public thought. In fact, Wellness continues to permeate into the public conscience even without advertisements or promotional campaigns of any kind. This is a necessary trait to have if a product, or in this case a lifestyle, has any hopes of lasting.

Continual Consumption

For a product or trend to last, that product or trend will continue to be in demand even after a consumer purchases it. In the case of Wellness, we can see this trait through items like vitamins or healthy food alternatives. Often when someone makes the switch to a Wellness lifestyle, that person will continue to commit him or herself to it by purchasing items necessary for dieting, exercising, and items used for preventive medicine.

Universal Appeal

Wellness affects not just a niche crowd or specified demographic but everyone everywhere. This creates a universal appeal, one that attracts everyone to the cause, no matter age, race, background, or gender. Wellness has such a massive universal appeal that going without it causes sickness and illness. Entrepreneurs see this as a prime opportunity to provide a much needed service to millions upon millions of potential consumers.

This universal appeal also makes Wellness one of the most sought after industries to enter into.

A Quick Consumption Time

In order for Wellness products to last in our modern economy and life, it has to be consumed quickly and in a relatively short amount of time and our society is one of 'go, go, go'. For a Wellness product or service to have any kind of lasting power, it must be accessed and enjoyed quickly.

These five characteristics all create something that will have a lasting power with the public. Products and services that promote Wellness must also have these five traits in order to hold their place in the minds of the consumers. So, it will be important for you, as you consider entering into the Wellness industry, to consider if the product or service you wish to promote, sell, or make available possesses these characteristics.

In the end, whatever field, product, or service you choose to have the most opportunity for your situation remember this,

Wellness is here to stay and it is important to enter the field now while it is still fresh.

The Wellness movement is pervasive; dare I say contagious? When we see a neighbor or friend enjoy the benefits of a healthy lifestyle, we are prone to want to imitate that change. This makes Wellness a "must have" which drives more and more consumers to seek products and services that promote healthy living and positive lifestyle changes.

For example, let's say that Mrs. Jones started going to yoga and began to eat nutritious snacks instead of chowing down on potato chips and sitting on the couch all day. You see Mrs. Jones one day and notice that she looks happier, leaner, and has a nice healthy glow about her. When you find out what she's doing, you decide to try it, you start going to yoga, eating the same healthy snacks, and as you feel the difference that a few lifestyle choices make, you begin to make more and more changes moving steadily towards Wellness. If you were the one with the yoga studio you would have gained one more client. If you were the one distributing the health snacks you would see an uptick in demand.

What Has Made Wellness So Desirable?

You may be asking yourself why Wellness is so sought after. Despite the obvious benefits of health and feeling good, why is Wellness such a desirable market to enter into?

As explained already, Wellness is more than a trend, it is a lifestyle change, one that people commit to for a lifetime. That alone makes this field attractive, especially for those wishing to start a business. Let's take a quick look at what first created this modern need for Health and Wellness.

Our society moved away from true Wellness decades ago with the advent of quick and easy meals and technological advancements that made many tasks in life easier. Instead of walking to work, we simply drive. Instead of pushing a hand mower to cut the grass, we sit in style and comfort driving a gas fueled mower. All these seemingly minor changes to how we do things have created a society of perpetual laziness and demand for the fast, the easy, the here and now.

There are a few factors that help to contribute to the modern day need for a strong Wellness industry.

Economy and Health

Obesity is a serious issue that is gaining attention every day. Over 65% of the population in the United States is obese. This is a dramatic increase from decades ago before the advent of fast food, laziness perpetuated by modern technology, and processed prepackaged meals that contain more salt than nutrition.

There now exists a new discrimination, one that is perhaps more powerful and more pervasive then race, color, or gender;

that new discrimination is based on wealth and health. Many look at the morbidly obese and equate them with poverty while the super wealthy are often nothing more than a stick and twigs.

Centuries ago obesity was a sign of wealth and privilege. Think about Henry VIII—he was a very fat and very rich man. Obesity is no longer a sign of wealth, it is now just the opposite, a sign of poverty. Why is this? It seems counter intuitive to me.

Remember that our current society works on a premise that responsibility can and should be avoided at all cost, that receiving a reward immediately is more valued then putting off gratification in favor of the better, healthier choice. This thought process leads many consumers to choose the quick and easy over the healthy alternatives. Why stand in the kitchen creating a healthy meal of noodles and seasoned baked chicken when you can easily run out to the store for a prepackaged microwavable meal or, if you are really lazy, ride to the fast food joint and go through the drive thru lane for a nice greasy burger and salty fries. The home cooked meal is obviously the healthier choice, but millions fail to make the healthy choice, instead opting for fast food and microwaved dinners.

This leads many to a life of illness, obesity, and a cycle of bad choices. The disparity between health and wealth is only perpetuated by our current disease based healthcare system where only the richest of the population can enjoy the benefits of physicians and adequate treatment for ailments and harmful conditions. This leaves low income individuals unable to treat the ailments and conditions that occur due to their continued bad lifestyle choices while the rich and wealthy are able to receive treatments and needed medication to counteract a bad diet and poor choices.

Being overweight and unhealthy has an incredible detrimental effect on that person's life, not just how they are viewed by others. Every facet of life from finding a job, to forming lasting relationships and even having enough energy to participate in everyday activities is negatively impacted by obesity and poor health. And, if you are unable to treat those conditions through quick fixes and remedies you are viewed as poor and uneducated.

Even if you are within the accepted weight range you are still more than likely unhealthy, due to poor diet and malnutrition. Malnutrition is not just a malady that is reserved for third world countries. A staggering number of U.S. citizens are more than likely suffering from malnutrition.

Of course due to our disease based healthcare system, where profit trumps health and Wellness, the population is told to accept the effects of malnutrition, headaches, fatigue, and stomach ailments as ordinary and to just take two pills and continue on.

Junk Food and McDiets

One of the most heinous crimes committed by the food industry is targeting low income families with junk food and unhealthy products. These processed foods, from fast food joints to snacks, are almost entirely sugar with a few hard to pronounce chemical names in the mix, have absolutely no nutritional value what so ever. While it is up to the individual to make healthy and safe food choices, there is a disparity when it comes to education about Wellness and preventive medicine and advertisements for sugar based, greasy, salty, food.

What's more, these foods are chemically designed to have a potato chip effect on your body so you cannot eat just one. If you ate a few apples or a banana or two you will soon move on to another type of food, maybe a carrot or an orange. But you will find it hard to be satisfied with just one fast food burger or a few fries. After a few days of eating these burgers and fries you will find yourself actively craving these harmful food products. To say that junk food and fast food joints sell their consumers addictive products is not going too far. In fact, this is in many ways similar to the way the tobacco industry engaged in business for years until legislation moved to curtail such actions.

Wellness products then should be designed to take advantage of this by offering healthier, easy alternatives to harmful foods and diets. Many restaurants are actually offering healthier menu alternatives but many of these establishments are offering too little too late.

The Sickness Industry

For the medical industry and healthcare field there is much money to be made when people are sick. Understanding how the current healthcare system works will go a long way in helping you establish a presence in the Wellness market and industry. Part of the modern Wellness movement is altering how we view healthcare. Our current healthcare is driven by profit instead of the well-being of patients. Almost every sector of the healthcare industry is driven by profit motivated by keeping you sick.

The current line of thinking for much of the medical industry is that we are sick due to bad genes or perhaps even bad luck. In reality it is our lifestyle choices that often determine if we get sick. It is time to realize this and work toward change. As you change your attitude and lifestyle; you will then be able to help others to change.[13]

Let us take a look briefly at the pharmaceutical industry and how their desire for a quick profit dictates the treatments you receive. Often the medication you receive may not be the best possible medication available. It is at the discretion of

---

[13]   Chestnut, p. 164.

your physician which medication to prescribe to you. Now, this is not always the case, and yes there are ethical doctors and pharmaceutical companies that do actually have your best interest in mind.

However, more than likely you are at the physician's or doctor's office due to a malady resulting from a poor lifestyle choice. That constant headache you suffer from and are seeking relief for may be the result of a condition that could have been prevented through an adherence to Wellness. Maybe you are too stressed or have a poor diet, whatever the reason, that headache can be prevented through good lifestyle choices and a commitment to Wellness. By changing your habits you can then eliminate the need for medication.

This means that stress reduction activities such as massage, yoga, and even acupuncture can have amazing results when applied to your headache. Prescriptions do not come cheap, which is leading many patients and consumers to what they see as alternative preventive treatments. Of course, these alternative preventive treatments have been employed for centuries by other cultures and are, in fact, Wellness programs that are proven to work.

The Baby Boomers are especially vulnerable to raising prescription rates even with the help of government agencies and programs. In an effort to reduce their need for medication and to save some much needed dollars, Baby Boomers are looking toward preventive medicine and care.

In turn, Generation X is seeing the Baby Boomers struggling with these prices and failing health and is actively seeking ways to improve their own health. They are finding more and more that true Wellness and Wellness products and services are the way.

Now, this is not to say that America's healthcare system is so bad off that it hurts more than it helps. Preventive care and Wellness, however, makes more sense so you can avoid unnecessary medications and hospital trips all together.

Wellness and the Answer to Our Health Crisis

There is now a need for healthier alternatives to the more traditional treatment options that we have been conditioned to deal with. Instead of seeking treatment after the onset of disease, much of the population is seeing the benefits of preventive medicine and care.

This has created a need in the market place ripe for the picking for those that have enough foresight to participate in the opportunity. There are several areas of the Wellness industry that one can benefit from both health wise and monetary wise. Remember, venturing into Wellness by establishing a business or taking advantage of an opportunity will result in helping those truly in need through education and providing them with affordable and available Wellness products and services.

The key then is to identify where in this new industry exists the potential for the greatest amount of growth. This will give you a notion of where to invest your efforts and money to gain the optimal return and thereby where you can do the greatest amount of good.

There are three primary areas of the Wellness industry that you can harness for your own business: Wellness insurance, Wellness foods, and Wellness medicine.

Wellness Insurance and You

To see the opportunities present in Wellness insurance you should first understand where the current insurance policies offered by employers have failed. By understanding this you will be better able to educate customers and direct them where their money can be better spent on their Wellness and preventive medicine.

The current disease based healthcare system is paid for almost entirely with health insurance. This system is valued at $2 trillion and is expected only to increase. This $2 trillion accounts for $6,667 annually for every single person in the United States, including you. That breaks down to $27,000 per year for a family of four. [14]

---

[14]   Pilzer, Paul Zane. *The New Wellness Revolution: How to make a fortune in the next trillion dollar industry.* New York: John Wiley & Sons, 2007, p. 132.

The current health insurance model, based on employers providing insurance to their employees is failing. This is because the cost of implementing the insurance continues to exceed profits for many businesses. What is more, the cost of insurance keeps rising at a faster rate than projected profits.

A new system of health insurance is beginning to grow in popularity, thanks to its ability to save the employer and employee money. What is being understood by those employers who are adapting the new insurance system, is that Wellness is really the only solution to the out of control costs of the current outdated and expensive health insurance model.

The current way the health insurance companies work is by trapping both employers and employees into a vicious cycle. They are then able to take advantage of these two parties to the fullest extent. Let's take a look at this scenario.

Illustrating the Problem

Say you work for Harlo Inc., a small company with just over 100 employees that offers health insurance. Over the course of your time with Harlo Inc. you develop a chronic disease (one that might have been prevented if you had practiced Wellness.) While you are still able to work you are now costing your insurance company thousands and thousands of dollars in medical expenses due to your condition. As a result the employer suffers a hike in their insurance premium, an increase that they are not necessarily able to handle.

This presents a serious dilemma to the employer. They now must shoulder increased rates due to your condition yet they are unable to outright fire you. And now because of your condition you must put in more hours at your job just to cover the added expense, while you are suffering as a result of your disease. You cannot quit your current job at Harlo Inc. to search for a job that offers more money or better coverage because employers are hesitant to hire employees with preexisting medical conditions for fear of increased premiums. And to top that, you will be hard pressed to find, let alone afford your own health insurance because, frankly, you will not be able to afford a plan that is not employer-sponsored because you have a preexisting medical condition.

Should you lose your job and are unable to find coverage privately you will soon find that many medical professionals will outright refuse to even make an appointment to see you. And if a doctor agrees to see you, that office visit is going to cost you well over 100% of what it might have if you had insurance.

This is why so many people wait until conditions and ailments are threatening their quality of life or every day activities before seeking any kind of medical help, usually through Emergency room visits.

Just by this scenario, which is faced every single day by an untold number of people, we can see how insurance companies benefit from the disease based healthcare system. They make more money when someone becomes sick; with rising premiums and other expenses they are then able to charge. Without insurance, clients cannot seek adequate care which forces many to pay those rate increases.

The reason for this is that many companies and businesses are only asking for insurance coverage that focuses on providing enough treatment to get that employee back to work. This goes back to the whole purpose of a disease based healthcare system which is to treat the symptoms and not cure the disease.

It has only been recently, within the last few years or so that employer-sponsored health insurance plans are beginning to cover preventive care options such as weight loss programs.

What is Wellness Insurance?

An alternative to the current insurance system is Wellness insurance. Wellness insurance works on the assumption that the individuals or families that purchase it will work towards being and remaining healthy thus eliminating the need for costly medical procedures, medicines, and other treatments that are only available to them once they have become sick or ill.

Wellness insurance covers the amount that is spent by these individuals and family groups for preventive care and medicine. This means that expenses used on vitamins, supplements, exercise programs, and the like will most likely be covered in whole or in part by a Wellness insurance program.

The idea is that by being proactive and adhering to a life where Wellness and preventive care is the focus, instead of living a life of bad lifestyle choices and throwing all caution to the wind, the amount of insurance claims will decrease. This deduction will result in lower premiums.

By being proactive about your health through Wellness programs you can reduce your risk for serious ailments later in life such as heart disease and diabetes. Such ailments cost insurance companies, and those they cover, potentially thousands of dollars, certainly enough to bankrupt many families each and every year.

Wellness insurance then rewards those covered by it by potentially eliminating the need for costly procedures caused by diabetes, heart disease, and obesity. This in turn saves providers money because they will not have to bear the burden of paying for procedures needed to treat such conditions and ailments.

The Individual Insurance Policy vs. Employee Sponsored Policies

One of the greatest benefits of an individual health insurance policy that is based on Wellness, and not simply on treatment, is that if you become sick and are unable to work you will not lose your insurance. Well, you will not lose it as long as you are able to pay your premiums.

With health insurance policies provided by employers you can lose your job and then your insurance if you become too sick or develop a condition that causes you to be unable to work.

With individual Wellness insurance, you are able to search for a provider that offers the lowest premiums. Premiums and rates are based on preexisting conditions and the likelihood of conditions developing. Insurance companies are then able to offer lower rates to those who are actively participating in Wellness programs.

Not to mention that when you are responsible for your own insurance you are going to take careful consideration of the rates and conditions offered by the provider. You are also going to take your own health more seriously since it is your money on the line should you fall ill or develop a serious medical condition.

We can already see some companies are offering Wellness insurance programs but for the most part it is up to the individual to find the right insurance provider. This presents a fantastic opportunity to you the entrepreneur. There exists a gap where people are seeking out professionals to educate them on proper Wellness insurance and/or Wellness insurance providers.

What You Can Do For Your Wellness Customers

By properly educating Wellness customers about alternative insurance policies you will find that they will save hundreds of dollars. The money they save will more than likely be invested into Wellness companies and services. This is because once an individual experiences the benefits of Wellness; they are eager to continue that feeling and to even amplify it.

Wellness insurance is based on remaining healthy and being proactive about potentially harmful conditions. The best way to do this is by continuing a life dedicated to Wellness. If you happen to have a business or are invested in the Wellness industry you will then benefit from the money that consumers are saving from seeking out individual health insurance policies.

This is similar to that vicious cycle created by employer-based insurance companies and the disease based healthcare system where the employee is trapped by the insurance terms so as not to risk losing coverage altogether. An individual insurance policy based on Wellness is a cycle in itself but of an extremely positive nature. In order to maintain their insurance they must also maintain their health.

By purchasing a Wellness insurance program the individual can expect lower rates if they are actively pursuing good life style choices such as weight loss programs and other preventive medicine and care. If the individual fails to adhere to Wellness programs and, say, starts smoking; they can be subjected to insurance rate hikes. In order to avoid such rate hikes many will choose to remain healthy because they are able to directly benefit from the decision of Wellness.

The individual will need to understand the ins and outs of Wellness insurance. Below I have listed a few important points that your potential customers will need to know about.

High deductible health insurance policy or HDHP is an insurance policy that has a high deductible and a lower premium but also offers certain Wellness benefits. For healthy individuals a HDHP is a great investment.

In order to have a HDHP you must also have a Wellness Savings Account (WSA). The WSA is an account that is opened at the time of purchasing the HDHP to hold the money you save from this kind of insurance. Normally, you will keep the amount of the deductible in the WSA to cover any medical emergencies or illnesses that may occur.

In order to be successful in any business that centers around Wellness, it is generally a good idea to begin in a field in which you have some experience. If you are knowledgeable about the insurance industry, then investing in Wellness Insurance is a logical step. Of course, if you specialize in, say, advertising then starting some kind of Wellness Insurance company is probably not going to be the best of ideas.

There are plenty of other areas of Wellness that you can venture into if Wellness Insurance opportunities are simply not your forte.

The Importance of Food and a Proper Diet

Remember that a major part of Wellness is proper diet and food full of nutrition. As a result, there is a huge available market in these fields. Today, not too many of us really understand what makes up a proper diet. We are a people bred on processed foods and sugary treats.

Before you start to invest into the Wellness food market, take time to review what food actually is and what a proper diet consists of.

What is This Thing Called Food?

For many of us, the only real requirement we have when it concerns food is taste. While taste is an important factor to consider, it is certainly not the only one. However, the food industry has created the thought that taste trumps all; therefore, if it does not taste great then there is no real merit in it. In actuality we need food for more than simply tasting great.

Food is fuel for our bodies. An improper diet has devastating effects on our bodies. A proper diet is one that has positive effects on our minds and bodies. When we are suffering from a diet of fatty foods and overly salted products we are sluggish, dull, and are afflicted with stomach cramps, fatigue, and headaches.

Food serves three primary functions: energy, catalyst, and building blocks.

The energy provided by food is received through calories needed to allow the body to function. Without the proper foods, internal organs like the heart and lungs will cease to function at peak performance. Many health problems can be traced to the body not receiving the proper amount or type of energy.

Catalysts needed by the body can be found in enzymes and in vitamins. These chemicals help to break down food and convert it into energy. Without enough proper catalyst components; we will soon find our body unable to properly process the food we eat. When this happens, we will soon find that everything from our mind to body is unable to adequately perform day to day tasks and leading to fatigue, aches, and other medical maladies.

The raw materials that are found in food, such as proteins, are necessary to create the human body. Our hair, nails, organs, skin and practically everything requires these building blocks and food is our primary source for it.[15]

Our bodies are designed to need these three traits and when we fail to receive an adequate amount of proper food and energy; we feel sick. Many of our day to day complaints about health can be traced to an inadequate diet.

To compensate, our bodies begin to crave foods with the highest amount of energy possible. These foods happen to also be

---

[15]   Hoffman & Deitch, p. 239.

the most delicious and are high in fat. For this reason many food companies create products that are high in fat and are delicious, tricking our bodies into believing that they are healthy and that we need them. This leads to the rising obesity and heart disease as well as the other ailments that are common in a lifestyle that features a poor diet.

We can then pinpoint two major problems with the U.S population and food. First, the majority of us eat way too much and secondly what we eat is not healthy.

Before you read any further, consider these three things that you can do right now to move toward Wellness:

1. Water, water, everywhere. Drink more water.

2. Eat fruits and vegetables. Many of us do not get enough fruits and vegetables in our diet which is shame since they are delicious and nutritious.

3. Supplements. The need for vitamin supplements and other forms are a great way to give our bodies a little extra help towards health. Supplements are also a great opportunity for those wishing to get into the Wellness market.[16]

---

[16]   Hoffman & Deitch, p. 251.

The Problem With Overeating

One of the most difficult hurdles to overcome on a path to Wellness is overcoming the urge to eat, eat, eat. Over half of the US population is overweight and there is really no end in sight unless there is a dramatic change in how food is perceived, manufactured, and marketed.

Until then it is up to people like you who understand the necessity of Wellness, and are seeking to enter into the Wellness market to lead the march to healthy eating.

Healthy eating is a habit that is going to be hard to form for those that are not already accustomed to it. What happens instead is that we just eat what is available no matter how healthy or unhealthy it is. Our stomach growls, we realize we are hungry, and we grab the first readily available items to chow down. Most of the time, that readily available item is high in fat and the human body stores fat in order to process carbohydrates. When your intake of fat gets too out of control; your body begins to store fat in easily visible places such as your stomach, thighs, and hips.

Think back to our ancestors; roaming the ancient land, spear in hand searching for food. Back then humans ate each meal as if it would be the last one for some time. This made sense, food was scarce but then humans developed agriculture and methods of preserving food. Now each meal is not our last yet many of us still eat like it is.

SELVA SUGUNENDRAN

Eating quickly does not allow our bodies to register the calories we are devouring. So our body keeps saying 'Feed me! Feed me!' Taking time between bites or courses will allow our body to process what you just ate and you will soon find that you were not as hungry as you might have thought.

Vitamins and Other Healthy Food Items

One of the leading causes of malnutrition in the United States and in other highly developed countries is the lack of food variety. This lack of variety leads many of us to miss crucial vitamins and minerals that we need in order to live a happy and healthy life.

Our bodies need vitamins, minerals, and proteins in order to successfully maintain our bodies and our cells. Without these crucial components our bodies and even our minds will begin to break down. It is easy to identify when you are not receiving enough vitamins. Mood swings, fatigue, headaches, muscle weakness and even certain cancers, and quite possibly Alzheimer's disease, can all be caused by a lack of essential vitamins, proteins, and minerals. The key is to listen to your body and live a life of Wellness.

Our current food supply offered on the major consumer market does not meet the nutritional requirement of our bodies. This does open a market place for vitamins and healthy foods that offer consumers the needed nutrition. Educating the public about appropriate sources of crucial vitamins and proteins presents another opportunity. Thanks to misleading advertisements by certain food industries the American public has the wrong notion of where they can get good protein and what products offer the best source of vitamins.

The Economics of Food and Opportunities For Wellness Business

Competition can be blamed for the current state of our food industry. Decades ago as technological advancements allowed food to be manufactured quickly and easily, businesses were competing with one another to see who could sell the most. In an effort to do this, manufacturers focused only on the taste of food adding more and more fat to make the food being produced appealing to our taste buds.

Unfortunately, knowledge about vitamins and nutrition was not up to speed with the ability to manufacture food. Basically, no one knew that just consuming mindless amounts of fatty foods was going to be detrimental to health so the only concern of food manufacturers was turning a profit.

What is worse, the process used for preservation and storage of food actually destroys vitamins that were once naturally in that food. This creates a system of food manufacturing that really has little to no nutritional value for those who consume it.

There is then a fantastic opportunity for you to offer the population a way to purchase healthy foods. Foods that are not overly processed, injected with preservatives, and packaged in such a manner to only offer taste and nothing of nutritious value. Healthy food is not bland. Healthy foods can be flavorful, robust, and amazing. All you have to know is how to offer these alternatives to the consumer.

The quest for Wellness is growing and as a result more and more consumers are looking for products that will aid them on their way to ultimate health. Food is an important factor in everyone's life and one of the most crucial elements to a Wellness lifestyle.

By offering products that are delicious and rich in nutrition you will be able to take advantage of what food manufacturers of the past missed. Food is more than food. Food is the building blocks of our bodies and eating properly is the key to living a healthy and happy life.

Wellness, Food and You

As Wellness continues to take center stage, these same food manufacturers are going to correct the various mistakes they have made in regards to how they manufacture and produce food items. If you are thinking about starting a business in this area of Wellness, the time to act is now in order to remain on the ground floor and to make the most out of this situation.

There are two areas where you will be able to find opportunities in Wellness food. The growing, harvesting, and transporting of foods and the education of consumers about healthy food are areas that are high in demand yet have very few businesses and individuals capable of meeting that demand.

Many attribute the failings of the U.S. government to the current state of the food industry. Now, the government did not fail the American people due to any kind of malicious intent but through outdated programs. Take the U.S. Department of Agriculture (USDA), which was created to protect farmers and their income. The USDA was established during a period of the U.S. history when farming accounted for a large portion of the country's economy. Now that number has dwindled as we look to other countries and regions from which to import food. The USDA, however, has not changed to adapt to the new shift of economy and instead of focusing on making sure the food we receive is healthy and nutritious, continues their outdated mission.

Outdated programs that are harming our food supply can easily be seen through agricultural subsidy programs.

What Are Subsidy Programs?

Ever since the Great Depression, American Farmers have been the beneficiaries of government subsidies.

An Agricultural Subsidy is a subsidy paid by the government to farmers as well as agribusinesses to (i) Supplement their income, (ii) Manage the supply of agricultural commodities and (iii) Influence the supply and cost of the relevant commodities.

Some examples of such commodities are cotton, milk, rice, wheat, peanuts, sugar, tobacco, oilseeds like soybeans and feed grains (i.e. grains used as fodder that includes barley, corn, maize, and oats).

But these programs have had an unfortunate and perhaps an unintended effect—rather than keeping the American public healthy, they have in fact contributed to the current obesity pandemic and a whole series of nutrition deficiencies. It is often argued that these policies have indeed encouraged obesity at the expense of desirable nutrition practices.

These policies have encouraged farmers to produce the most subsidized crops such as wheat corn and soybeans. It has therefore compelled farmers to ignore crops such as fruits, vegetables and other grains.

The result of all this is that the supermarkets are flooded with products derived from highly subsidized crops, such as sweeteners, in the form of high fructose corn syrup (HFCS) hydrogenated fats derived from soy beans, and feed from pigs and cattle. The direct effect of this is that the prices have dropped dramatically for unhealthy and fattening foods such as ready to eat meals, prepackaged snacks, corn-fed pork and beef as well as sweetened soft drinks. The result is that the healthier alternatives are relatively higher priced due to either no subsidy or poor subsidy. This explains why obesity is so prevalent among poor people who could only afford the cheap obesity-causing food.

Barry Popkin, a professor of nutrition at the North Carolina has stated that, "We put maybe one tenth of one percent of our dollar into what we put into subsidizing and promoting foods through the Department of Agriculture into fruits and vegetables."

It is also argued that the decline of prices of unhealthy foods account for as much as half of the increase in obesity. In effect what happens is that "people face cheaper food and they eat more and they weigh more."

Richard Atkinson, a professor of medicine says, "If America is going to subsidize agriculture, the least it could do is to subsidize healthy foods. There are a lot of subsidies for the two things we should be limiting in our diets, which are sugar and fat, and there are not a lot of subsidies for broccoli and Brussels Sprouts. What would happen if we took away the subsidies on the sugar and fat? Probably not much. But if we are trying to look for something political that might make a difference, try subsidizing fruit and vegetable growers so the cost is comparatively lower for better foods."

Benefits of Small Farms vs. Corporate Farming

The rapid and dramatic increase of factory farming or Industrial agriculture has made it extremely difficult for the small farmers to remain in business in the United States. Unfortunately their increase is accelerated by government policies that favor large scale production. The result is very few young people become farmers today.

The argument put forward by the supporters of corporate farming is that if industrial farming results in more food at a lower cost, doesn't that benefit consumers

If food was like the mechanical parts used in machinery, it might make sense. But where the health, environment and community life is disrupted by mass food production, then the way the food is produced and transported matters as much as what is in the food itself.

Today just a few corporate food manufacturers are determining what is made available to consumers in the supermarkets. In this situation, shouldn't consumers find out where the food originated so that they could decide on the choices they make

As health is so dependent on the food we eat, it is important to examine why the small farmers are important:

(i) Local farmers produce fresh, nutritious and high quality foods.

(ii)   Small farmers live on or near their farms, they have a vested interest in natural resources and human health and so do not indulge in the industrial agriculture operations which pollute communities with noxious fumes, excess manure, and chemical pesticides.

(iii)   The existence of family farms also promotes the preservation of green space, local employment and trade within the community.

(iv)   Small farmers maintain the diversity in our food supply

(v)   Local farming encourages families to cook fresh food and vegetables instead of eating fat, sugar and preservative-based food that has travelled an average of 1,500 miles.

(vi)   Small farmers use border cropping, sequential and crop rotation, while corporate farms use monoculture, leading to empty niche spaces.

(vii)   Foodborne diseases are prevalent in corporate farming foods such as fruits and vegetables that get contaminated with pesticides while hormones are added to milk.

(viii) The so called traditionally safe and nutritious foods coming from small farmers are not that safe when they come from corporate farmers. The dangers include, cancer caused by pesticides, contamination from x-rays used to remove bacteria from food, ecoli and salmonella. excess antibiotics used on animals are also being investigated for harmful results in food.

By encouraging Corporate farming, the government has increased the availability of processed foods which provide a higher fat and calorie content. Our yearly per capita consumption of sugar has increased from 128 to 158 pounds and average calorie content by 10%. The result is that Obesity is a major problem in our society as doctors have classed 3 out of 5 children as overweight with a possibility of diabetes at 1 out of 3.

This has created two areas of farming and agriculture that need to change in order to meet the modern day demands of Wellness consumers:

- Which foods the farmers produce; and
- How these foods are produced.

And, production should be through organic means.

Right now most farmers are bound to subsidy programs when deciding what to grow and harvest. This means that they are unable to listen to consumer demands and what the market actually wants. Wellness farmers, on the other hand will be able to grow what they want and how they want, meeting market demand and filling a gaping hole in the agriculture industry.

Right now many farmers are forced to grow food that they do not want to grow based on subsidy programs which, in most part, is based on what corporations are demanding in an effort to push those foods onto consumers. Often these foods are not as healthy as advertised. Milk, for example is healthy but not in the quantity that we were led to believe.

With proper education about Wellness and health many consumers will instead switch to healthier alternatives to cow's milk, such as almond based milk or soy based milk.

It is all about proper education for the consumer and then creating products and services to provide for the consumers.

The Soy Example and the Opportunity For Wellness

Soybeans were not well known a few decades ago. And to be honest not too many people outside of the Wellness movement really give soy much thought. The fact is that soybeans present an amazing opportunity for the business entrepreneur. This is because soy is healthy, less expensive to produce, and is incredibly green. Despite the fact that the United States produces 50% of the world's supply of soybeans, the average American will have no idea what a soybean looks like let alone how it tastes. [17]

Soy has been used for thousands of years in many Asian countries. Like with other Wellness products and practices, we in the West are only now starting to catch up to what has been known for centuries by those in the East. The soybean is a great source of protein and, unlike other protein sources, is low in saturated fat and has no cholesterol. Soy also contains several vitamins and minerals needed by the human body to perform simple everyday tasks.

The true benefits of soy are only now being explored. Just recently the FDA has explored the health benefits of soy and its role in a proper diet. Soy has been shown to lower certain diseases and conditions such as heart disease. This means that soy and soy based products are an excellent source of Wellness and preventive medicine. By adding soy to your diet, one can reduce the risk of heart disease while lowering cholesterol levels. Soy can even help those with diabetes since it slows the rate of digestion and the speed at which foods are absorbed into the body.

There are plenty of ways to add soy into your diet:

- Soy milk which can be used on its own or as a substitute for milk in recipes and for sauces.

---

[17]   Pilzer 2007, p. 85.

- Soy protein powder can be used instead of flour in many baking recipes.
- Soy protein powder can be sprinkled on breakfast cereals.
- Soy can be substituted in meat based dishes such as tacos or burgers.

The uses of soy are only limited by one's creativity. It is easy to see how lucrative an industry based on soy can be, yet the United State sill fails to ingest an adequate amount of this protein despite its proven benefits.

While soy is no longer a food known only to the most extreme of vegans and vegetarians, there still exists a need for affordable and widely available soy products in the market place.

An Example of a Successful Soy Business

The benefits of soy as a healthier alternative to meat and milk cannot be argued. It is evident in the research and the effects of a soy based diet on an individual's Wellness and health. You may be a bit hesitant though about starting a business in the soy industry, especially if you are a first time entrepreneur. This is understandable, for many people soy is still a mysterious product suffering from various misconceptions about its taste and texture. The truth is that soy is delicious and when substituted into recipes, is virtually indistinguishable from what it replaces.

Steve Demos is an example of what kind of successful business opportunity soy represents. Demos started White Wave, Inc. in the mid 1970's with the goal to create tofu and other soy based products. He wanted a viable and sustainable product that not only tasted great but was healthy as well. Many of these products were actually way before their time and did not do so well at the time of their introduction. However, SILK managed to have a lasting effect in the market and is still found in nearly every major grocery and food retailer today.

SILK is soy based milk and offers all the great taste of cow's milk without any of the negative drawbacks. SILK managed to make an impact in the market because it so closely resembled cow's milk.

Soy Milk is a dairy free beverage that is similar in texture and taste to cow's milk. One of the main benefits of Soy Milk is that it is created from a vegetable source. The extracted milk is often fortified with Calcium and Vitamin D in order to increase its nutritional value.

Since Soy Milk has no cholesterol, it is an excellent option for those suffering from heart diseases. According to FDA, Soy Milk proteins in fact reduce cholesterol.

Since Soy milk is created by vegetable proteins it contains no lactose and therefore is suitable for individuals who are lactose intolerant.

Soy Milk is rich in isoflavones which, in addition to reducing cholesterol, eases the symptoms of menopause, prevents osteoporosis and even potentially reduces the risk of prostate and breast cancer.

Here is an "at a glance" short list of comparison of Soy milk vs. Cow's milk.

(i)   Cow's milk has twice the fat of soy Milk.

(ii)   Casein, 80% of protein in cow's milk, is a mucus-maker.

(iii)   Soy Milk's Fiber content compares with "NIL" in Cow's Milk.

(iv)   Soy Milk has only 25% of salt content of Cow's milk.

(v)   Soy Milk has the necessary amount of Magnesium to make 100% of Calcium useable but milk has only 12% of the necessary Magnesium.

(vi)   Pasteurization kills vitamin "D".

(vii)   A cup of whole cow's milk has the cholesterol content of 17 slices of bacon. Soy Milk has none.

(viii)   8% of Fat in Soy milk is Omega 3 while 50% of the fat is Omega 6—both essential fats.

White Wave saw a 37% increase in 1997 shortly after launching SILK. By 2004 White Wave saw $362 million in sales led mostly by their SILK product. [18]

The opportunity for success in soy products is certainly not limited to soy milk. For the ingenious and innovative, marketing and manufacturing soy based food products can result in extremely lucrative returns.

Ultimately, people want to be healthy and once the full extent of soy and similarly healthy products is known beyond the Baby Boomers and those select groups already keyed into the Wellness movement, there will be no limit to the demand of healthy food products.

Restaurants and Wellness

As the population begins to focus their thoughts on Wellness and start to make the necessary changes to accommodate that new way of life, they will not be too keen on giving up certain luxuries that they have come to enjoy. Eating out is enjoyed by nearly every single family in the United States today and accounts for 45.6% of a family's food budget. [19]

---

[18]   Pilzer 2007, p. 89.
[19]   Pilzer 2007, p. 96.

Decades ago the thought of eating out at a restaurant was only reserved for special occasions or for the very wealthy. Now, there are restaurants and fast food joints on nearly every street. Restaurants line downtown districts and fast food establishments dominate highways and shopping districts.

Everywhere you turn you are going to find some place offering some kind of cuisine whether it is French, Chinese, Thai, or Mexican. These places cater to every lifestyle and schedule, form fast food establishments for the busy family on the go while sit down restaurants cater to those who have a little extra time on their hands.

What is missing is a restaurant solely dedicated to offering healthy alternatives. Sure, some establishments are starting to alter their menus to offer healthy choices but there are very few places that are dedicated to offering a menu centered on Wellness.

Those entrepreneurs who are looking to enter into the Wellness industry are now presented with a fantastic opportunity; that of offering healthy menus at restaurants focused on Wellness. As Baby Boomers contemplate their health and turn to Wellness, they will be looking for products and services that cater to their new lifestyle. Unfortunately for them there are too many restaurants focused on Wellness. Fortunately for you, this means that there is a perfect opportunity ripe for the picking.

You may be wary about this opportunity, wondering how many people would flock to a restaurant to eat healthy food, instead of zipping through that fast food drive thru to pick up a quick and easy burger loaded with fat and grease.

Decades ago, before the restaurant industry picked up any significant steam of clients, entrepreneurs of the day were hesitant about investing in the field because food preparation was so expensive. Not only this but there was not enough potential employees to man the restaurants and the consumers simply lacked the time to go out and eat.

This all changed as technology progressed and developed in such a way to drive down food manufacturing prices. This same technology also eliminated some jobs and their employees turned to the restaurant industry as a source of employment. As life got easier and more efficient and the work day shortened; families found that they had more free time to go out and enjoy a bite to eat.

This same trend is going to happen within the Wellness restaurant industry. As more and more consumers demand healthy food and Wellness products, the cost of these products will decline as competition increases. With the uptick of demand for healthy foods, the restaurants and fast food establishments already in existence will either be forced to make quick and dramatic changes or close their doors all together. By acting quickly on this opportunity you can get your foot in the door and establish your restaurant, or service, or product as a quality Wellness alternative.

On Wellness, Medicine, and Opportunity

The opportunities available for Wellness medicine are not going to be solely restricted to those already in the medical field. In fact many of the recent innovations with Wellness and medicine have come from people that have never had anything to do with the medical field. These people managed to see a gap in how healthcare worked and decided to take advantage of that gap.

Hippocrates, the famous Greek physician and the name sake for the Hippocratic Oath, was a pioneer of his day. He was the first to focus on treating the body as a whole and not in segments, separate from each other. Hippocrates was certainly the first to work on preventive medicine and care. He understood the importance of a proper diet and exercise, with the understanding that sickness was not a normal state.

Somewhere through the course of history modern medicine has lost sight of this. Instead of focusing on the body, mind, and spirit as a whole, medicine divides the physical from the rest and focuses only on treatment. The modern medical perversion of Hippocrates' findings and studies has resulted in untold damage to patients for centuries.

As medical science advanced doctors and physicians have gained greater understanding of the human body. Now, in the modern day, we are able to understand the building blocks of life itself and what is needed to make those building blocks

SELVA SUGUNENDRAN

function properly. To the surprise of many, Hippocrates was right. Prevention is the best way to combat disease.

Hippocrates recommended the flowing Wellness program for optimal health:

• Exercise

It is hard to get enough exercise throughout the day especially in our modern society, but it is crucial that you get enough physical activity.

• Vitamins

It is important to get enough vitamins and supplements. This ensures that your body is getting the required protein to function properly and to keep your mind sharp. It is commonly agreed upon that there are four supplements that are a Wellness must. These supplements are: Fish Oil, Vitamin D, Probiotic, Micronutrient Formula (make sure it is a certified organic whole food micronutrient).[20]

• Calories

Our bodies need the proper amount of calories to provide fuel for basic functions such as growth, digestion, and to avoid weight gain.

• Avoid Chemicals

Harmful chemicals used to preserve packaged and processed foods are not natural. As a result these chemicals can have detrimental effects on the human body and should be avoided.

---

[20]   Chestnut, p. 265.

Opportunities in the Wellness industry then offer entrepreneurs the ability to learn from Hippocrates' Wellness outline. This means that the vitamin and supplement industry is ripe for entrepreneurs that are willing to take the risk, with the understanding that Wellness consumers are going to be looking to vitamins and supplements as a way of replacing what they are missing in their food supply.

One such entrepreneur was Carl F. Rehnborg, who developed the Nutrilite Company. Rehnborg noticed that people living in urban areas in China were suffering from malnutrition yet citizens in rural areas were not. The same was true for many areas of the world.

He developed the idea of a product that combined the vitamins an individual needed into an easily consumed item. This product was distributed by salespeople that traveled the country educating consumers about the need for vitamins and selling the multivitamin. The salespeople were able to hire additional salespeople and were even able to draw income from their sales.

This helped to create Nutrilite as the leading source of multivitamins.

The key here is that Rehnborg saw that there was a need that was created by modern food manufacturing. That need was to restore the vitamins and supplements individuals were lacking.

Opportunities abound in the Wellness medicine field. Through the distribution and sales of vitamins and supplements, you will be able to reach those individuals that are ready to change their life for the better through Wellness. You can even work to educate these individuals on the proper use of vitamins and why we need them. Education is the key to change and by properly educating consumers on the need for vitamins and supplements, you will quickly attain customers for life.

In order to find a successful product to sell, that product must be needed and must be consumed on a regular basis. While this model is used by the disease based healthcare industry to ensnare patients into buying prescription drugs, the difference is that vitamins and supplements are healthy and go toward preventing sickness instead of perpetuating it.

Where Knowledge is Power

Knowledge is a commodity in itself and in an industry that is still relatively new to the masses, it is a highly prized commodity. One such company that understood the need to provide knowledge about Wellness products to the masses is ConsumerLab.com.

This site was founded with the intent of providing information about vitamins and supplements to the masses. Regulation is lacking when it comes to many supplements and as a result many unscrupulous manufacturers take advantage of consumer ignorance. These manufacturers provide subpar and even harmful products to consumers.

As a result, many individuals are left with the idea that all vitamins and supplements are either harmful or simply fail to work. Ask yourself, do you believe that vitamins work to improve health? If not, then you were probably one of the victims of unethical companies peddling poor quality vitamins.

Common problems with these vitamins and supplements are:

- These vitamins or supplements contain harmful chemicals.

- These vitamins simply do not contain what they are supposed to.

- These vitamins fail to release their ingredients because of a poor manufacturing process.

ConsumerLab.com took it upon themselves to test vitamins and supplements for the consumer market. The company then rates the products and provides a description about the product and how well it works.

For consumers this knowledge is invaluable.

In this scenario, ConsumerLab.com provided consumers not with new technology but with information. This information is invaluable for the consumer wanting to make the best possible decision about their Wellness. Information and knowledge is just as valuable as Wellness products and services like yoga, exercise, and meditation.

Without accurate and honest assessments of Wellness products, like vitamins or supplements, the consumer will never achieve any state of actual Wellness. If you want to get into the Wellness industry but lack any kind of manufacturing ability, you can always invest in educating consumers about Wellness.

Wellness is still a relatively new movement and consumers tend to shy away from ideas and products they perceive as new or strange. Education is the key to demystifying the concept of Wellness for potential customers. By enlightening the masses about Wellness, you will create a strong customer base.

The Potential in Exercise

There are many opinions on how much exercise one needs. The question often asked is," Surely there must be an optimum amount of exercise?"

To be quite frank, the answer depends on who you ask, as you will see below:

(i)   Taiwan Study on Health & Exercise: Fifteen minutes of exercise could add 3 years to your life.

(ii) UK Health Department: Everyone should aim for 150 minutes of exercise per week which averages to 21.5 minutes each day of the week or 30 minutes five days a week, which is the generally recommended schedule.

(iii)   Centers for Disease Control and Prevention (CDC): Thirty minutes a day for good health.

(iv)   NICE: Thirty minutes of moderate exercise at least 5 days a week. Moderate exercise includes walking, cycling and gardening.

(v)   Human Performance Lab: Forty-five minutes of vigorous exercise is good for weight loss. This type of exercise impacts the metabolic rate for 14 hours. You could lose up to 500 calories during exercise and another 250 calories during the next 14 hours. This means a person wishing to shed a great deal weight may do 45 minutes of exercise at (say) 6am and then again at 8 pm and could potentially lose around 1,400 calories. This could translate to around 140 pounds in a year.

(vi)   Harvard Medical School: A test was carried out on women, with an average age of 54 years, and concluded that those who gained weight later on in life found it more difficult to lose weight through exercise alone. But they also concluded that 30 minutes a day of exercise prevented many health problems but did not result in much weight loss.

In conclusion, we will say 30 minutes a day is good but for weight loss you may need to try the exercise routine as set out by the human Performance Lab. In any case it depends very much on your current health condition and you should always consult a medical practitioner.

Entrepreneurs like you can do well by looking into implementing exercise programs and fitness clubs. The need for exercise cannot be understated. By creating an area where people can exercise in safety and in peace is important to help promote Wellness.

Finding the time and place to exercise is a hard task, especially in this modern age. Potential clients want a place to exercise that is conveniently located and equipped with not just the most up to date equipment but the most useful as well.

Opportunities in physical exercise exist in many areas not just establishing fitness clubs. Fitness trainers, massage therapists, and chiropractors are all needed in the Wellness industry. The opportunity exists to employ these professionals in private practice or by establishing a Wellness center.

Wellness presents many opportunities for the savvy investor and entrepreneur. The key is to possess a desire to make money and to help people by promoting Wellness.

Take a careful look at your skills and abilities and decide which area of Wellness you can serve. If you can create a database of vitamins and supplements as well as their benefits then why not create a company designed to provide this knowledge to customers? If you are able to provide training in exercise, then why not start your own personal training business?

The point is that you have an unlimited amount of opportunities in the Wellness industry. Just ask yourself where you can do the most good, while still making a profit.

Finding business opportunities in Wellness medicine does not require you have any prior medical training. All you have to do is find a gap in the market where there is a legitimate need, either for vitamins and supplements, knowledge, or physical exercise and then consider how you can turn that gap into a viable business.

Sounds hard? Well, let's take a look at some of the other ways you can make money through the Wellness industry. Just remember that entering into a new business is a scary prospect. You are taking a risk, but rest assured that the Wellness industry is not some trendy fad that is going to go out of vogue next season.

Everyone, from grandma to your babysitter, wants to be healthy and one of the best ways to achieve that state of being is through Wellness. Of course, there are other ways of providing Wellness to the masses while making a profit.

The Distribution of Wellness

Those who are interested in making money (and who isn't?) probably know by now that the "secret" to success doesn't necessarily lie in imitating those who have already made a fortune, but rather in finding a strategy that, while based in the same fundamental principles, will work for you and your particular strengths and interests. So far, this chapter has talked about the potential of cashing in on the Wellness revolution by understanding the need for high quality products and working to develop and manufacture those products (such as supplements or Wellness-promoting foods). However, it is plain that this is not everyone's forte. Even if this is the case with you, do not despair, there are still other opportunities through which you can make your fortune in Wellness.

Consider, for instance, what might be possible if your core business strength lies not in creating and developing, but rather in selling. Being good at selling products is a strength that the Wellness revolution sorely needs, because without such people providing this valuable service, the average person will never be aware of the availability of these Wellness-promoting products and how they could change his or her life. In other words, even though manufacturing is a vitally important part of business, it is nothing without distribution in place to get the products to people who wish to purchase them.

In fact, it has been written that distribution may well be the more critically important side of the coin in this matter. If nothing else, it is the easier discipline to master, and the one over which people tend to have more direct control. Those who develop products for sale are ultimately at the mercy of market trends; they must anticipate the next major trends that will occur within a particular consumer demographic and then develop products that will appeal to that trend in a high quality way. On the other hand, distribution is a more consistent effort. While the nature of distribution does change over time, the truth remains that it is fundamentally less volatile than manufacturing, such that consistent success can be achieved simply by focusing on distribution and "distributing the ever-expanding production of cutting-edge technology". [21]

In other words, you need not develop or create products yourself to make a fortune in Wellness; you can simply choose to distribute cutting-edge products that others have already made, providing that you do so smartly!

Unlimited Wealth

In order to understand that distribution can generate a fortune for you without your own personal investment in development or manufacturing, it is important to understand a key economic principle. Economist Pilzer wrote about this principle at length in his work, "The New Wellness Revolution", where he called it the principle of "unlimited wealth".

---

[21]   Pilzer 2007, p. 167.

SELVA SUGUNENDRAN

The basic idea is that we live in a society where people tend to specialize in one thing, and then make that one thing their career. This works because, as we do something over and over, we get more efficient at it, and tend to produce higher quality results. Over time, the work we do increases in value and generates greater returns on investment. For example, if you're in the business of selling, you probably don't sell paper on Mondays, wheelbarrows on Tuesdays, telephones on Wednesdays, shoes on Thursdays, and children's toys on Fridays. Instead, you have a particular niche where you know the products exceedingly well and are effectively able to communicate the value of these products to clients that are interested in buying them. As people tend to specialize in any one area of business, the profit potential in that area of business increases exponentially, and unlimited wealth is attained, at least in theory.

There is, sadly, one major bottleneck to unlimited wealth, and that is distribution. If someone was particularly good at selling paper, such that the majority of sales opportunities they engaged in resulted in a sale, that person should be able to make a fortune. Their ability to do so is limited, however, by the number of sales opportunities in which they can engage. Indeed, as Pilzer writes, "the total overall wealth of a society is thus limited only by distribution."[22]

---

[22]   Pilzer 2007, p. 168.

It should be plain, then, that if you, as a sales-oriented person, can find new and exciting ways to expand distribution in a specialized way, then you too will be able to vastly increase your profit potential in connection with the new Wellness revolution, even if what you're distributing is someone else's products. So, by all means, if sales and distribution is your forte, embrace it!

The Secrets Behind Distribution

To truly generate the most value from your sales efforts, however, you absolutely must understand the fundamental philosophy behind the practice of distributing products. Indeed, distribution is not simply a physical exercise in getting a product from point A to point B. If it was, then there would be little profit incentive here, as that particular service is already well provided for by organizations such as FedEx, United Parcel Service, and the post office. While physical distribution channels are an important part of making a profit through distribution, an equally important part is also educating the public about the availability and desirability of the product in question. As you well know, you may have access to the most innovative and valuable product ever seen in the Wellness industry, but unless you can communicate the need for that product to clients, you aren't going to be able to sell a single unit.

SELVA SUGUNENDRAN

Therefore, in order to profit through distribution, you must pay a great deal of attention not only to how you're going to physically distribute the products in question, but also how you're going to get the word out and demonstrate the value of the products to as many clients as possible.

At first, this may seem like a daunting task, but the payoff is definitely worthwhile if you're willing to take such an effort all the way. To see the wisdom in such a statement, all you need to do is take a look around at the condition of the market in the last few decades and ask yourself who the biggest success stories are. Sure, there are a few entrepreneurs who made their fortunes through the development and manufacture of some core technology, like Apple's Steve Jobs. However, the vast majority of people who have made their fortune in the last few decades have done so not through developing and manufacturing the most innovative products, but through distributing those products to the public. For instance, the "geniuses" behind Google, one of the most compelling success stories of the digital age, made their fortune not by creating the millions of websites that Google indexes and serves up to users every day, but simply by finding a way to raise awareness about those sites and distribute them to users (via search engine) in a way that was compelling and highly useful. Google didn't even develop the fundamental search engine technology, which had been around nearly a decade before they started using it, they simply refined it in such a way as to maximize both the education and distribution sides of the equation. Additionally, successful online retailers such as Amazon.com have managed to generate a considerable amount of wealth not by making innovative products themselves, but through making these products available to the public via an innovative and compelling distribution format.

Indeed, trends are moving in such a way as to favor distributors over manufacturers. To see the truth of this, one need only look at how physical retailers have changed over the last few decades. It used to be the case that the most successful retailers were specialty shops and department stores. However, that is now changing, such that the most successful physical retailers are "big box" mass merchandisers like Wal-Mart, Costco, and Target.[23] Think about what this signifies for a moment. Generally speaking, these companies certainly don't have the same high quality of goods and services that specialty stores or high end department stores do, but they are nevertheless dominating the marketplace. This speaks to the importance of distribution. Often the product itself is of secondary importance to the means used to distribute it to the public.

In order to compete with these entities, an all-new species of retail entity has emerged into the marketplace: the category buster. This refers to a company that engages in "mass merchandising in one category of goods."[24] For example, Lowe's

---

[23]   Pilzer 2007, p. 173.
[24]   Pilzer 2007, p. 175

SELVA SUGUNENDRAN

is a category buster that focuses all of its efforts on distributing home repair and renovation supplies. Staples or Office Depot are category busters in the field of office supplies and paper goods. The lesson here is clear. If you don't have the resources to be a wide-scale mass merchandiser who provides competent and effective distribution of a whole category of Wellness-related goods, don't worry about it. Instead, simply focus on a single category of Wellness goods that you CAN effectively promote and distribute, and the results will be just as good. It's all about specialization.

Say that you love to cook, so you know more about the availability of fine high-quality Wellness ingredients than anyone else involved in the Wellness industry at the moment. This may be your cue to make gourmet Wellness foods your specialty category. The same holds true if you're into nutritional supplements and know all about them. Anytime you can truly and passionately communicate the value of a product to your clients, that may well be a product you should be selling, as it's one you'll be able to effectively distribute.

Zero Marginal Production Costs

While passion plays a major part in effective sales, and especially so in an industry like Wellness, it is unfortunately not the only consideration which a profitable distributor of goods must keep in mind. In addition to selling what you know and love, you should also seek to sell those items which you can make the most money on per unit.

Let's say, for example, that you're all about Wellness foods. At a convention, you happen to hit it off with a Wellness-minded chef who makes and packages his own gourmet whole-grain ravioli, made with the finest whole ingredients. The two of you briefly discuss matters and agree to try out a scenario in which you distribute the locally made ravioli through your national distribution pipeline, as a re-seller, if you get a volume purchasing discount from the chef. Let's say then that you have to pay $2.00 for each package of ravioli you stock, you spend another $3 on distribution costs, and sell each package for $8. That's a total of 3$ profit on each unit sold.

On the other hand, let's say you meet a Wellness-minded supplement developer who makes a supplement with locally made ingredients that are not readily available in the rest of the country. You make the same reselling agreement with her. Because of the abundance of the ingredients in the local region, you are able to acquire a bottle of the supplement for just $.50 and it costs you $2 to distribute. Then, because of the scarcity of the ingredient elsewhere in the country, you're able to charge a premium rate of $10 a bottle, which people gladly pay. The profit on each supplement sold is then $7.50, or more than twice the profit you make on the ravioli. Even though your passion is Wellness food and you're more personally interested in the ravioli than in the supplement, it only makes sense that you would place more sales emphasis on the supplement, due to the higher return on investment and profit potential.

The reason this is so important in this day and age, has to do with yet another principle of business that helps to further explain the success of mass merchandisers. even further. For some goods and products, the total cost of production for each unit can be reduced to virtually nothing. This is a total maximization of profits, in that any money one makes from reselling such a product is pure profit, as the sheer volume of sales and offerings has reduced the cost to virtually nothing.

If you put in the time to do the research, you'll find that this is particularly true for many of the products sold in the Wellness industry, especially foods and supplements. All you need to do is look around until you find products that you, in your unique individual circumstances, can distribute for virtually zero cost. This will give you a powerful key advantage in that category of Wellness sales, at which point you, just like the majors, should bust that category with all your emphasis and sales power.

Direct Selling

Of course, it should also be mentioned that the price at which you can sell goods is not determined entirely by circumstance or by the original developer or manufacturer. Indeed, there are certain things which a distributor can do to cut costs sharply, simply by modifying the method through which the product is distributed. Far and away, the most popular method for reducing costs, both for the distributor and consequently for the end user, is "direct selling". Direct selling refers simply to selling products directly to the client through some interface, either person-to-person, or in more recent times, via a website, that is in some ways the opposite of simply stocking a store and letting clients come to you. There are many who chastise direct sales for being "outdated" in this day and age when people are said to value speed and convenience over demonstrated value, but this is simply not true. In 2005, more than 100 billion dollars were raised through direct sales alone.[25] Moreover, it is estimated that at least 75% of the United States population still engages in purchasing behaviors through the direct sales channel.[26] So much for the idea that direct selling is dead.

When you engage in direct selling, it has the benefit of allowing you to carefully control the costs of everything you sell. You have very little overhead, it costs you nothing in itself to "stock" merchandise, and your product pipeline is very straightforward, flowing from the manufacturer to you to the end user. For this reason, your only real costs are the cost of the item itself, and the cost needed to distribute the item. There is nearly always

[25]   Pilzer 2007, p. 191.
[26]   Pilzer 2007, p. 191.

SELVA SUGUNENDRAN

something you can do to trim away at either of these and still turn a profit. This allows you to maximize the profit value of each item you sell through your direct sales approach.

Direct Selling and Residual Income

Another major benefit of direct sales is that it can bring you a good deal of residual income. It must be stated, for the record, that there are two key types of income with which you must be concerned if you really hope to make a fortune in any market, much less the Wellness market. Active income is income that you receive directly in response to some labor that you carry out. For instance, if you mow someone's lawn as a kid, and receive $20 for the job, that's direct income. To get another $20, you're going to have to find another lawn to mow. Now let's say you grow up to be a famous rock musician (congratulations!). You write a hit song early in your career, and a month after the album comes out, you get a nice fat royalty check for thousands. That might be considered direct income as well. However, the next month you'll get another check for royalties on that album, assuming it continues to sell. If you've written a real hit, you may still be getting royalty checks years into the future. Even if you never write another song besides that first hit, it can continue to generate income for you long past the initial effort you put into it. That is residual income, and how people truly get wealthy. [27] Of course, it's not just for artists and rock musicians. You can earn residual income off of stock investments, books that you write, and, most importantly to this chapter, Wellness goods that you sell through direct selling!

How does this work? It's quite simple. Recall that we've established that distributing a product really consists of two actions: the first is the education of the client that the product exists and that they need to buy it, and the second is actually getting the product to them. The first can be difficult, but the second is nearly always a breeze. However, if you do a good job of direct selling, you're not just moving product, but establishing long term relationships with clients that will continue to pay well into the future. If you sell a client a supplement that really addresses his or her needs and changes his or her life in a profound way, that client will almost certainly continue to buy that supplement from you, month after month. This means that, just like the rock star, you put in the initial effort to demonstrate the value of the product, and then it leads to long-term residual income that pays off well into the future.

---

[27] Pilzer 2007, p. 194.

SELVA SUGUNENDRAN

Evaluating a Direct Sales Opportunity

Having explored how direct selling can be valuable to a distributor working in the Wellness industry, it is important to cover a few logistical points. For instance, how do you know what products to work with in your direct selling venture? In order to make this determination, it's necessary to engage in a little psychological exercise. Basically, you'll need to place yourself in the position of the client and ask some fundamental questions about the value of what you're selling—and most importantly, you'll have to answer truthfully. For any given product that you have the opportunity to sell, place yourself in the client's position and ask yourself if you had never heard of this product before now, would it be something that you would have an interest in buying? If you can't imagine yourself ever seeing the value in a product and wanting to buy it for your own use, you can't reasonably expect a client to see that value either. In short, if you wouldn't buy it, neither will the client. This means that, no matter how attractive a product might be in terms of price or cost, or no matter what sort of relationship you have with the manufacturer or developer, you should not attempt to sell it if it doesn't meet this "honest" evaluation. Otherwise, it will drag down your efforts to make your fortune in Wellness.

Another vital question to ask yourself, when determining whether or not you want to attempt to add a product to your direct selling repertoire, is whether or not the product really contributes to Wellness. To be sure, Wellness is the new emerging trend in health and like any trend, there are those who will respect the industry and treat it legitimately, as well as those who will attempt to treat the industry like a passing fad, something to make a quick buck at and then get out before it collapses. But as someone who knows something about health and sickness, as described in Chapters One and Two, you know that Wellness is not a fad. It is an enduring principle of human physiology that is not going to change anytime soon. Therefore, it is in the best interest of anyone who seeks to make a fortune in Wellness to respect the integrity of the industry and only sell those products which truly and legitimately contribute to the Wellness of clients. This requires the use of your common sense, as well as a working knowledge of what health and Wellness really are. A product that makes extravagant claims and promises to promote Wellness but in fact does little for the client may well net you one sale, and while that may be enough for the fly by night entrepreneur, it's not enough for the entrepreneur who really wants to work in the Wellness industry and make a fortune. Those of us who are in it for the long-term, demand products that really and truly contribute to the Wellness of a client and improve their quality of life on a fundamental level. This is what makes it all worthwhile. This is what generates the loyalty that produces lasting client and seller relationships and, in turn, residual income from those same loyal clients who order month after month. If your product does not truly seem

SELVA SUGUNENDRAN

to contribute to long-term Wellness, it is not worth your time to sell it. Move on.

It's also worth mentioning at this point that some direct sellers choose to work for a direct sales organization, rather than pick and choose their own products from developers and vendors that they personally seek out. This can have its advantages and disadvantages. The primary advantage, of course, is that one has to put little effort into finding products and goods to sell; one simply sells what is available through the organization and collects the profits therefrom. One may also have access to a wider variety of higher quality merchandise this way, depending on the organization for which one works. However, there are some major disadvantages that you should look out for as well. For instance, most of these organizations charge some sort of fee. At times this fee is totally fair and offsets the greater ease with which products are available and won't really cut into your profits because of the higher volume that you can move, but at other times, it can be exorbitant and make the whole endeavor hardly worth your while. Sometimes these organizations can exhibit predatory behaviors that are not really in the best interests of direct sellers, but rather exist primarily to make a profit for the owners of the organization. In short, the quality of direct sales organizations differs wildly, and if you're going to work for one, you had best be sure that it's a legitimate organization that offers what you're looking for before you cast your lot with them.

Luckily, there are some guidelines you can use to make such a decision. As Pilzer points out in his book, the Direct Sales Association offers a set of guidelines in the form of a "Code of Ethics" that all forthright sales organizations should follow. [28] If the organization you're considering working for does not meet these fundamental criteria, the odds are good that in the long run the working relationship is not going to work out the way you expect. Think long and hard about joining any such organization, and be sure to look out for the following characteristics:

- **Start-Up Costs**

A high quality direct sales organization will want to forge new relationships with sellers, and will thusly have few barriers to entry. The start-up costs associated with joining will generally be quite low. This is because well-established functional sales organizations have the confidence that a seller will be around for the long term and allow the company to profit that way. However, a fly by night organization that hopes to exploit sellers knows that sellers aren't going to stick around for long once they realize what's going on and consequently they want to charge as much as possible upfront so that they can make all the profit they can before the sellers run away. Consider high start-up costs a dire warning sign about the quality of any sales organization.

- **Options to Purchase**

---

[28]   Pilzer 2007, p. 197.

A high quality sales organization will recognize that products sell differently in each region, or that sellers will have unique specialties and be better able to sell one type of product than another. As such, they are all too happy to let sellers pick and choose what products they wish to try and sell, and allow sellers the option to purchase products or not purchase products. Again, they adopt the long-term view that allowing a seller to grow his or her business organically is better for long-term profits than forcing a seller to adhere to some rigid guidelines that aren't going to work for everybody. If an organization requires you to sell certain products that you aren't sure about, think twice before joining up.

- **Fees**

The bottom line, in regards to fees, is that a high-quality direct sales organization will only charge you money based on the products that you sell. The more products you sell, the more of a fee will go to the company, because they take a small percentage from each sale. This is a fair deal, and the way it should be, because it means that both the company and the seller have an equal interest in getting products sold. Unscrupulous sales organizations, however, generally require sellers to pay certain fees regardless of whether or not they actually sell anything. The problem with this is that the company has no incentive to actually help promote and facilitate sales. Once they hook the seller, they're already making a profit off their fees, so they could care less whether the seller is actually able to get the products to an end user or not. Inquire upfront about the nature and quantity of fees before joining any sales organization.

- **Return Policy**

Lastly, a high-quality sales organization will allow you to return unsold inventory after a period of time. Everyone makes mistakes in the sales business, but they need not be catastrophic. Suppose that you over-estimated the value of a particular product and ordered much more of it than you were able to sell. After having several crates of Blopco's Wellness Enhancer EX-4 sitting in your garage for a year gathering dust, you realize that you've made an error and won't be making your money back on that particular product. If your direct sales organization is upfront, they will recognize the problem and generally allow you to return the products in question, for at least some percentage of the price you paid. A poor direct sales company has already made their money off you, however, and they have no incentive to play ball so they'll refuse to buy back the unusable product and you'll end up stuck with merchandise that's going nowhere.

Opportunities in Wellness Insurance

At this point, we should bring up the topic of a particular type of Wellness product that goes beyond the standard fare of equipment, supplements, and food: Wellness insurance. As mentioned in the first chapter, the healthcare system in the

United States is largely based around the idea of insurance. The cost of healthcare is so extravagant that no one can afford it outright; rather, people pay premiums to an insurance company that will then foot the bill if you get sick. In effect, it's gambling against yourself. Health insurance is getting more and more costly, and more and more people are uninsured which is a major reason why the Wellness revolution has arrived and this is also a powerful selling point for the Wellness entrepreneur.

People are already acclimated to the idea of paying for health insurance. However, they are rarely satisfied with their insurance and the coverage it provides. This means that you, as a Wellness entrepreneur, have the unique opportunity to educate the individual about the benefits of Wellness insurance. Rather than betting on the fact that they will get sick in the future, they can take their health into their own hands, develop a healthy lifestyle and promote a sense of Wellness that will drastically reduce their chances of ever needing to use the health insurance they're paying for.

The idea behind Wellness insurance is that people reduce their payments on health insurance to purchase term policies, and invest the difference into a Wellness program that minimizes their chances of ever needing that insurance in the first place. This still offers one protection, but it also fundamentally improves the quality of one's life, which is something that cannot be said about traditional health insurance.

In other words, selling Wellness products and services is actually a form of insurance. Framing it this way for the client, can help them to make wise decisions about their future and demonstrate the real value of what you're selling.

Use What You Know

The above is but one example of how a seller can use the skills and experience they already have from their current careers to supplement their efforts to profit from the Wellness revolution. Be prepared to use what you know to develop a niche for yourself in this market and succeed beyond your expectations.

For instance, if you have experience with farming, perhaps you can begin to devote a segment of your crops to Wellness-promoting foods and begin to educate your clients about their value. If you're a retailer, you can undertake a similar educational campaign through selling and actively promoting products in your retail space. Those involved in the health industry, such as nurses and therapists, can help their clients even more by actively promoting the idea of Wellness instead of just perpetuating the same old cycle of sickness-based "health". Use your imagination and explore what skills and talents you have that can be an asset in the coming revolution.

CONCLUSION

In the end, Wellness is one of the most significant trends to impact the state of healthcare in the United States in the history of this country. Trends have advanced to the point where our current sickness-based system is simply no longer sustainable. Patients, doctors, insurance companies, in fact no one, can continue much longer with our current system. And why should they? As shown in the first chapter, the current system is going nowhere fast and we're putting more money into a system that is giving us all less and less in return.

The bottom line is that something has to change, and that something is the focus of our healthcare system. Instead of focusing on how to recover once we get sick, we're going to have to start focusing on how to stay healthy in the first place. All across the country people are getting motivated to take their healthcare into their own hands and make wise decisions about their lifestyles that are geared toward promoting long term health.

As they do, they'll be changing their dietary habits, their lifestyle choices, and along with those, their purchasing habits. This means that the Wellness revolution is a powerful opportunity for the insightful entrepreneur. By knowing what purchasing decisions Wellness-focused people are going to make, today's entrepreneur can get in on the ground floor of a revolution that will pay dividends far into the future.

Because you now have insight from this book, there is positively no reason that you can't be one of these people! You can make your fortune in the Wellness revolution, and, at the same time, help make this a better world through improving the lives of your clients. All it takes is a little understanding of what Wellness really is, and a committed desire to help people achieve that Wellness in the best way possible.

Thank you for reading, and good luck with wherever you decide to take your Wellness career, from this point on.

Long live the revolution!

To our health!

CPSIA information can be obtained at www.ICGtesting.com
Printed in the USA
LVOW061005100713

342103LV00002B/119/P

9 781479 735051